D1238362

INTERNATIONAL SERIES OF MONOGRAPHS ON
PURE AND APPLIED BIOLOGY

Division: **ZOOLOGY**

GENERAL EDITOR: G. A. KERKUT

VOLUME 21

THE COMMON LIVER FLUKE

A

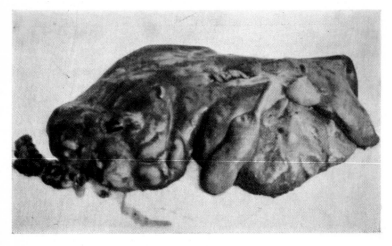

PLATE I Bovine liver damaged by *Fasciola hepatica*
(Photograph by permission of the Controller H.M.S.O.)

The
Common Liver Fluke

Fasciola hepatica L.

BY

E. M. PANTELOURIS

Department of Zoology
The Queen's University of Belfast

PERGAMON PRESS

OXFORD · LONDON · EDINBURGH · NEW YORK
PARIS · FRANKFURT

Pergamon Press Ltd., Headington Hill Hall, Oxford
4 & 5 Fitzroy Square, London W.1
Pergamon Press (Scotland) Ltd., 2 & 3 Teviot Place, Edinburgh 1
Pergamon Press Inc., 122 East 55th St., New York 22, N.Y.
Gauthier-Villars, 55 Quai des Grands-Augustins, Paris 6
Pergamon Press GmbH, Kaiserstrasse 75, Frankfurt-am-Main

First edition 1965

Library of Congress Catalog Card No. 63–21135

PRINTED IN GREAT BRITAIN BY THE BAY TREE PRESS, STEVENAGE, HERTS.

CONTENTS

Part IV

ECOLOGY AND CONTROL

PREFACE

THE liver fluke, *Fasciola hepatica*, causes great damage to stock throughout the world, and is responsible not only for "liver rot", the uncomplicated fascioliasis, but also (in association with the bacterium, *Clostridium oedematiens*) for the notorious "black disease". Moreover, numerous cases of human fascioliasis are reported each year.

To its economic importance should be added the great biological interest of a Trematode with a succession of free and parasitic generations, ending up in a physiological relationship with the mammalian host that presents a variety of important aspects for study; a Trematode moreover that has so far avoided radical control by man: drugs fail to kill its younger migratory stages, vaccines are ineffective, neither ecological measures nor grazing management eliminate all risk to stock (although they greatly reduce it), and many wild animals provide a reservoir of infection.

The liver fluke is therefore the concern of the zoologist as well as the veterinarian and agriculturalist. It is the aim of this book to provide: for the research worker, a thorough review of the extensive literature on the subject and a comprehensive bibliography, as well as practical details of techniques for handling material; for the veterinarian, biologist and agriculturalist, an account of our knowledge about this important animal and the disease it causes and of the way in which this knowledge has been accumulated.

The author is indebted to many for generous help with the work involved in writing this book. I wish particularly to thank Dr. J. F. Gracey, Professor R. A. R. Gresson, Dr. D. L. Hughes, Miss Barbara Knox, Dr. C. B. Ollerenshaw, Mr. T. Ross, Mr. A. W. Stelfox, Dr. L. T. Threadgold and Dr. J. R. Todd, who have discussed various aspects with me and have provided data and information from their work. Dr. Threadgold has taken the trouble to prepare original drawings illustrating his findings about the structure of the worm. My sincere thanks are also due to those who have helped in the search for the more inaccessible references or with translations from Hungarian, Japanese, Polish and Russian. Finally, I thank Miss Barbara E. Knox for checking the manuscript and Mr. S. Armstrong for expert photographic work.

E. M. P.

Zoology Department,
Queen's University, Belfast.

ACKNOWLEDGEMENTS

The author would like to acknowledge the helpfulness of publishers and authors who have given permission for the use of illustrations from their publications. In each case the source of the material is indicated by the reference quoted in the caption to the figure.

PART I

BIOLOGY OF THE LIVER FLUKE

CHAPTER 1

LIFE CYCLE AND SYSTEMATICS

THE common liver fluke, *Fasciola hepatica L.*, is a parasite flatworm that can be collected in large numbers from the bile ducts of infested cattle, sheep and other mammals. The infestation causes loss of condition, renders the liver unsuitable for human consumption and reduces the amount and quality of meat and milk produced. In severe cases the infestation may cause death either directly, or indirectly by initiating or aggravating bacterial infections, as in the case of "black disease".

In years when weather conditions favour the parasite, "liver rot" or fascioliasis (as the liver fluke disease is called) may assume the proportions of an epidemic and decimate flocks. It is, however, very difficult to assign a figure to the economic losses caused throughout the world by fascioliasis; no comprehensive statistics exist, much of the damage is indirect, taking the form of loss of condition and productivity of the animals, and the disease may be caused also by other similar fluke-worms. However, to indicate the size of the problem, a list is given of some relatively recent reports from various countries (Table 1).

Outline of the Life Cycle (Fig. 1)

The worms found in the bile ducts of mammals represent the adult stage of the liver fluke. They are leaf-shaped, about 30×10 mm, whitish or tinted. They are hermaphrodite and produce enormous numbers of eggs; these reach the host gut with the bile and are shed to the outside with the faeces.

By this time the egg contains an early embryo. Under favourable conditions, this develops further whilst still within the egg to form a conical larva, covered with a ciliated epithelium and equipped with a pointed tip or rostellum at its anterior end; this larva is called a miracidium.

TABLE 1. SOME RECENT DATA ON THE INCIDENCE OF FASCIOLIASIS.

Reference	Region	Period	Abattoir statistics (Livers condemned)		Estimates of incidence, mainly from detection of eggs in faeces		
			Cattle %	Sheep %	Cattle Infected %	Sheep Infected %	Deaths %
1	Anglesey	1958–59	63·3	15·3			12·9
2	Ireland, Northern	1946–54				38·6	
3	Scotland, Central	1958					60
4	Wales		29				
5	Devon	1954, June	17·7				
6	United Kingdom						
7	Poland	1951–52			50		
8	Lithuania	1956			91	46	18
9	Rumania						
10	Bavaria, Regensburg	1945	8·3				
10	Bavaria, Regensburg	1952	20·9				
11	Sweden, Ostergotland	1953	21·5				
12	Milan (Italy)	1960	35·5				
13	Netherlands	1957–62	10·3	19·1			
14	Rhodesia, Southern	1956–61	5·7	2			
15	South Africa	1951–57				15	
16	Japan	1958	68		40		
17	Japan, Higashimatsuyama	1952	7·5				
18	Puerto Rico		37·5				
19	U.S.A. Gulf Coast						
20	U.S.A.		2·6				

N.B. Data from various regions are not strictly comparable; for example, in most countries only the rather heavily infested livers are condemned, and the thoroughness of the inspection procedure may vary. The data assembled therefore in this Table serve to indicate the widespread incidence of fascioliasis and its substantial economic importance rather than to establish valid comparisons of incidence. Furthermore, incidence varies enormously from year to year depending on weather conditions.

1   Anon. (1959). Figure refers to ewes, 12,000 of which died in the epidemic that winter.

2   Data supplied by the Belfast City Veterinarian, Dr. J. F. Gracey. See also Table 19 and Fig. 62.

3   Parnell *et al.*; see Fig. 62. In a survey of "a typical hill sheep farm in the Western Highlands", Wilson *et al.* (1953) found 50 per cent of the ewes and whethers and 24 per cent of the hoggs infected.

4   Anon. (1959).

5   Peck (1957). Data from Hatherleigh knackery.

6   Peters and Clapham (1942). Data from 486 slaughterhouses (73,000 cattle).

7   Stefanski (1959).

8   Babenskas *et al.* (1958).

9   Lungu (1959).

10   Keller (1952).

11   Sallnäs (1954).

12   Carrara and Recalcati (1961).

13   Honer and Vink (1963). Survey of 3 largest abattoirs covering 710,401 lambs under 13 months old, January 1957–June 1962. See Fig. 63.

14   Condy (1962). Data refer to infection with *Fasciola gigantica*.

15   Purchase (1957).

16   Ono (1958).

17   Takashino *et al.* (1960).

18   Rivera-Anaya and De Jesus (1952).

19   Schwartz (1947).

20   Olsen (1949a).

On hatching from the egg, the miracidium rotates and moves in the water by the action of its cilia, but it can survive for only a few hours, unless it finds and enters a suitable snail host. If a snail of the species *Limnaea truncatula* is available, the miracidium is attracted to it and bores, rostellum first, into its tissues. In the process it loses the ciliated cover and elongated shape, to become a sac-like sporocyst.

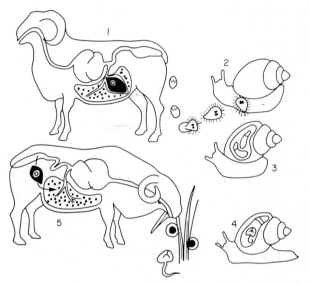

FIG. 1. Diagrammatic representation of the life history of the liver fluke.
1. The adult parasite in the bile ducts of a sheep; its eggs are shed on the pasture. 2. The ciliated miracidia hatching from the eggs enter a snail host. 3. The larvae have now formed rediae in the digestive gland of the snail. 4. The rediae have given rise to tailed cercaria. 5. The cercaria become free of the snail, encyst on the grass and the cysts are picked up by grazing animals. The cyst releases the metacercarium in the alimentary canal of the final host, and the young fluke migrates through the viscera to enter the liver.

As the sporocyst grows within the snail, new and different larvae develop inside it: the *rediae*. These are mobile and break free by rupturing the wall of the mother sporocyst. In favourable cases, the sporocyst finds itself eventually in the pulmonary cavity of the snail, but the redia migrates from there to the digestive gland or "liver" of the snail host.

Feeding on the substance of the snail liver, a redia gives rise to several daughter rediae. Each one of these may again repeat the process, growing and producing a further generation of rediae. Eventually, however, the rediae give rise to still another type of larva, the cercarium. This is round with a long unforked tail; it leaves the snail through the pulmonary cavity and swims free in water, finally attaching itself on to a blade of grass or other object; in the meantime it loses its tail and becomes a metacercarium enclosed in a cyst.

It is these cysts that are infective to grazing mammals who may pick them up with the grass. In the stomach of the mammal the metacercarium excysts, bores through the wall of the gut into the abdominal cavity and reaches the surface of the liver. It then bores into the liver mass and tunnels its way through it, feeding and growing, until, as a mature egg-producing adult, it settles in the bile ducts. In badly infested animals, tens or even hundreds of flukes can be found blocking the larger bile ducts. Their eggs reach the host's intestine with the bile, and are shed with the faeces, to begin another cycle.

To summarize, the life cycle of the liver fluke comprises several morphologically distinct stages; of these, both sporocysts and rediae are capable of multiplication, so that up to a few hundred of cercaria may eventually arise from a single egg. Two hosts are involved in this life-history, a snail and a mammal. The free larval stages are produced in large numbers but require moisture, and are non-feeding and short-lived.

The Discovery of the Life Cycle

The fascinating story of how this complex life cycle was elucidated has been told by Taylor (1937) and in more detail by Reinhardt (1957). Some points have been discussed by Jefferies and Dawes (1960).

The earliest references are listed by Schaper (1890), but the ideas then current about the liver fluke had little foundation on facts.

An idea of the prevailing explanations in those times may be provided by a quotation from a book of 1837 on Sheep Husbandry where it is stated about the liver rot: "It is caused simply by the extrication of certain gases or miasmata during the decomposition of vegetable matter, under the united influence of moisture and air." (Simmonds, 1880.)

However, in 1698 the Dutch anatomist, G. Bidloo, did write a 64-page essay on the liver fluke in the form of a letter to Leeuwenhoek. Noting the numerous eggs in the worm, he suggested that the mammals become infested by swallowing eggs with drinking water. Van Leeuwenhoek also, in some of his letters to The Royal Society (1700 and 1704), assumed that the worms enter grazing animals through the mouth, but could not explain why he was unable to find any liver flukes in samples of soil or water from pastures. Linnaeus had the rather incongruous idea that the fluke is a leech swallowed and modified in the host.

Towards the end of the 18th century it became recognized in certain quarters that some parasites divide their life-time between two or more hosts. Steenstrup (1842) developed the idea of an alternation of generations and actually dealt, among other groups, with Trematodes; he seems to have been aware of the larval stages only and not of the adult stage inhabiting the vertebrate host. Having described the rediae (which he calls "nurses") and the cercaria of Trematodes, he concludes that ". . . the species must, from the egg upwards, necessarily pass through several generations succeeding each other in a definite order before it appears as individuals which both externally and internally resemble those from which the course of development commenced and which are capable of propagating the species anew by the generation of ova" (from the English translation by Busk, p. 94). Cercaria, rediae and miracidia had been seen and described as independent forms quite early (by Müller, 1773; Bojanus, 1818, and Mehlis, 1831 respectively), but Steenstrup's new theory connected them together for the first time. Simonds (1852) showed that liver fluke eggs as such are innocuous to sheep. Confirming the presence of rediae in snails Weinland (1875) speculated that cercaria may encyst on grass.

All these facts and ideas paved the way for the unravelling of the life cycles of Trematodes such as the liver fluke, and for the identification of snail hosts. This was actually achieved under the impetus provided by the severe epidemic of 1879–80, when three million sheep were lost in Britain. Whilst Rolleston (1880 a and b) expressed the suspicion that the slug *Arion hortensis* might be the intermediate host, a young demonstrator in Oxford, A. P. Thomas,

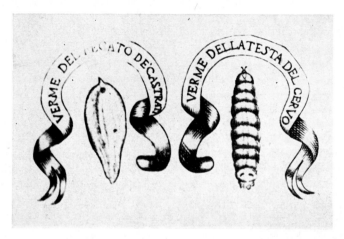

FIG. 2. An illustration from Francesco Redi's book *Esperienze intorno alla generazione degl' Insetti*, Firenze, 1668. The liver fluke is illustrated on the left and described as the *verme del fegato de' castrati*, i.e., the worm of the liver of sheep.

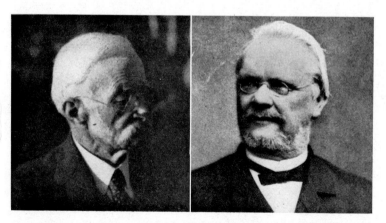

FIG. 3. Left, A. P. Thomas (1857–1937). Right, R. Leuckart (1822–1898).

B

was given a grant from the Royal Agricultural Society to investigate the problem. At about the same time, the problem was being tackled by Professor R. Leuckart of Leipzig. The two men worked almost in competition for priority. The results were two series of papers (Leuckart, 1881, 1882 a and b; Thomas, 1881, 1882 a and b; 1883 a and b) in which the snail, *Limnaea truncatula* was indentified as the host and the successive larval stages were bred and described.

The work of the two main pioneers was supplemented in essentials by Lutz (1892–3) who demonstrated the infectivity of the cysts; and by Sinitzin (1914) and others who established the route followed by the metacercaria from the gut to the liver in the definitive host.

Systematics

As already mentioned, the common liver fluke, *Fasciola hepatica* Linnaeus 1758 belongs to the phylum Platyhelminthes (the flatworms) and more specifically to its subdivision Trematoda. The Trematoda are considered usually as a class, and the Phylum is considered to comprise three such classes: the Turbellaria, the Cestoda and the Trematoda. Again, the Trematoda are usually subdivided into three sub-Classes (or Orders): *Monogenea*, a group comprising ectoparasites on the gills or skin of fish and other aquatic animals, with a simple life cycle and no second host; *Aspidocotylea*, endoparasites with a simple life cycle, and characterized by a large ventral sucker covering like a shield a large part of the body and often elaborately subdivided; and *Digenea*, endoparasites with a complicated life cycle involving several larval stages and from two to four hosts.

Whilst the above scheme is the one adopted by textbooks up to recently, it is now being superseded by a new one. Several authors, like Van Beneden in the last century, and Baer and Bylchowski at present, have drawn attention to the dissimilarities between Monogenea and Digenea. Bylchowski (1957) has devoted a monograph to the subject and has raised the Monogenea to a separate Class, implying a closer relationship of the Digenea to the Cestoda rather than to the Monogenea. In a recent textbook (*Traité de Zoologie*, P. Grassé editeur, Tome IV, premier fascicule,

Masson, Paris, 1961) the following scheme is adopted for the phylum Platyhelminthes:

Class 1. *Turbellaria*   Free, generally direct development.

2. *Temnocephala*   Ectoparasites on Crustacea and other fresh water animals, absent from regions over 40° latitude.

3. *Monogenea*   Endoparasites, unsegmented, parasitic mostly on fish, some on Copepods parasitizing on fish or on Amphibia and Chelonia. No second host.

4. *Trematoda*   See below.

5. *Cestodaria*   Parasites mainly of the gut of fish.

6. *Cestoda*   No trace of intestine at any stage.

The Class Trematoda more specifically is subdivided into three sub-Classes:

(a) *Aspidogastrea*, equipped with a single ventral adhesive disc subdivided by grooves into muscular segments; no suckers; endoparasites of fish, reptiles, etc. but with direct development.

(b) *Digenea*, endoparasites showing polyembryony in the first host.

(c) *Didymozoidea*, endoparasites of fish with direct development, especially adapted to living enclosed within the cysts formed around them by the host tissue.

The Digenea are further subdivided into two groups, one retaining the original excretory vesicle in the adult (*Anepitheliocystidia*) and the other with a secondary excretory vesicle in the adult (*Epitheliocystidia*). Further subdivisions into Orders and families may be based on the structure of the cercaria; this is considered by some a better basis than either structural characters of the adults, or the grouping together of forms parasitizing related hosts.

The genera *Fasciola* (formerly *Distomum*), Linnaeus, 1758; *Fascioloides*, Ward 1917; and *Fasciolopsis*, Looss 1899 make up the digenean family FASCIOLIDAE. *Fasciolopsis* can easily be distinguished from the other two, in that its intestinal caeca are simple and not dendritic. *Fascioloides* again shows no distinct cephalic cone, in contrast to *Fasciola*; and its yolk glands lie ventrally to the intestine, whilst in *Fasciola* they spread both ventrally and dorsally to it.

Most species of this family deserve the description "liver flukes" in that, at the adult stage, they parasitise the liver or the bile ducts of mammals or birds. All Fasciolidae are characterized by a comparatively large, leaf-like body which may be opaque, whitish or tinted; elaborately branching reproductive organs and intestinal caeca; and the position of the uterus which is small and coiled and lies anterior to both testes and ovary. Size differences of some species are shown in Fig. 4.

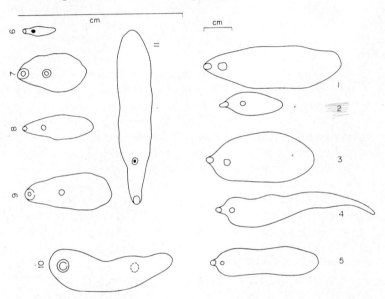

FIG. 4.   Diagrams to scale to show approximately the relative sizes of some liver flukes. 1, *Fasciolopsis buskii*. 2, *Fasciola hepatica*. 3, *Fascioloides magna*. 4, *Fasciola nyanzae*. 5, *Fasciola gigantica*. 6, *Dicrocoelium dendriticum*. 7, *Eurytrema pancreaticum*. 8, *Opisthorchis felineus*. 9, *Haplorchis sp*. 10, *Paramphistomum sp*. 11, *Clonorchis sinensis*.

There are still other liver flukes, belonging not to Fasciolidae but to related families: the small or lancet fluke, *Dicrocoelium dendriticum*; *Eurytrema pancreaticum*; *Clonorchis sinensis*; and certain species of the genera *Opisthorchis*, *Metorchis* and *Pseudonymphistomum* (Fig. 4).

The liver flukes affecting ruminants are: two species of *Fasciola* (*hepatica*, the common liver fluke; *gigantica*, the large liver fluke of

Asia and Africa), *Fascioloides magna*, the large liver fluke of America, and *Dicrocoelium dendriticum*, the small "lancet" liver fluke. There are also flukes living in the rumen (*Paramphistomum cervi, P. microbothrium* and *P. liorchis, Cotylophoron* sp.).

Species of *FASCIOLA*

It might be helpful to list here the other species of the genus *Fasciola*, not only because their life-cycles are similar to that of *hepatica*, but also because their separation as distinct species is often doubtful and a matter of some dispute among systematists.

Fasciola gigantica, Cobbold 1856, was at one time known as *Cladocoelium giganticum*. It is larger than *hepatica*, and the crural branches are more nearly vertical to the main branch of the gut; also the eggs are larger in comparison to those of *hepatica*. *F. gigantica* has a wide range of snail hosts. In Turkmenia, for example, larvae of this species were found in 32 per cent of *Radix lagotis*, 27 per cent of *R. ovata*, 34 per cent of *R. pereger*, 16 per cent of *Galba truncatula* and 10 per cent of *Physa acuta* (Kibakin, 1960); all except the last could also be experimentally infected.

The areas of distribution of the two species overlap partly. In Pakistan for example, Kendall (1954) finds *Fasciola hepatica* predominating in the highlands, and *F. gigantica* in the lowlands, with an intermediate zone where mixed infections are common. *Limnaea truncatula* is found only above 4000 ft and *L. auricularia* is probably the host of *F. gigantica* in the lowlands. Mixed infections are on record also from Thailand (*Disshmarn*, 1955). Similar overlapping of distribution of the two species but with undisputed prevalence of *gigantica*, has been ascertained also in Turkmenia (Kibakin, 1961), Japan (Watanabe, 1955; 1958), Turkey and the salt-marsh area of Armenia. In the latter, 97 per cent of fascioliasis in sheep is caused by *gigantica* (Davtyan, 1955).

Fasciola indica has been proposed as a new species (Varma, 1913), as being intermediate in character between *hepatica* and *gigantica*; Sarwar (1957), however, considers this as synonym for *F. gigantica*. Price (1955) considers it likely that the liver flukes prevalent in the Gulf Coast region of the U.S.A. are hybrids of *hepatica* and *gigantica*, the latter species having probably been introduced with Brahman cattle imported from India in 1875–1906.

In America, Ssinitzin (1933) claimed two new species which he named *Fasciola californica* and *F. halli*. He gives the following differences of these from *F. hepatica*: Host of the first is *Galba bulimoides* and occasionally *Galba bulimoides techella,* host of the second is *Galba bulimoides techella* only. The first has scales on the dorsal side of the posterior half of the body in the adult, whilst the second is covered with scales throughout and these are larger than in *F. hepatica*. Both species take 2 months to run through one life cycle.

Fasciola nyanzae, Leiper 1910 (Fig. 5) was studied recently by Dinnik and Dinnik (1961). Specimens were obtained from the

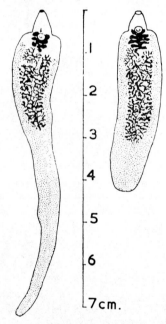

FIG. 5. On the right *Fasciola hepatica* and on the left a large specimen of *F. nyanzae* from the hippopotamus (Dinnik and Dinnik, 1961).

hippopotamus in Uganda. The yolk glands are located both dorsally and ventrally to the gut; the latter lacks the ramose internal diverticula of *gigantica*. The area occupied by the ramified testes is smaller than in *hepatica* and *gigantica*. Although no snails were found naturally infected, the aquatic species *Limnaea natalensis* could be infected in the laboratory. No rabbits or goats could be infected with metacercaria and it would appear that *Fasciola nyanzae* is specific to hippopotamus.

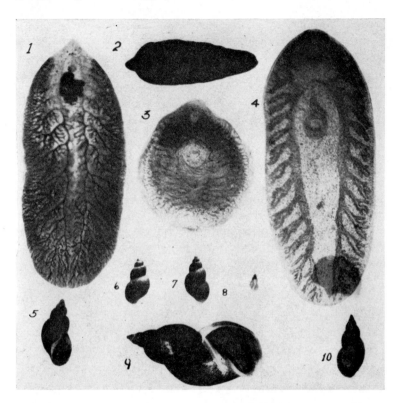

FIG. 6. 1. A specimen of *Fascioloides magna* from deer. 3, 4 — Young stages of the same species. 2 — *Fasciola hepatica* for comparison. 5–10 — snail hosts in Canada. 5–8 — specimens of *Fossaria parva*. 9, 10 — *Stagnicola palustris nutalliana* (Swales, 1935).

Another species, *Fasciola jacksoni* Cobbold, 1869, has long been known from the elephant and has been re-described recently (Bhalerao, 1933). The adult is 12–14 mm long and 9–12·5 mm wide, round or pear-shaped. The gut has crura both internally and externally to the two main branches. The testes are central and lie one behind the other.

Although in a different genus, *Fascioloides magna* (Bassi, 1875; Ward 1817) should be mentioned here as it is often the cause of fascioliasis in America. In fact, it was previously described as a species of the genus *Fasciola* under the specific names *F. magna, americana* or *carioca*. This fluke is a natural parasite of deer in North America, but occurs also in bisons, horses, cattle, sheep and goats (Fig. 6). In sheep and goats it causes severe symptoms, but in deer and cattle these are slight. In cattle, in fact, it is claimed that the adult worms are trapped in thick cysts in the liver and no eggs can be shed from the host. (Swales, 1935, 1936; Griffiths, 1962). This incidentally makes the parasite inaccessible to anthelminthics.

In a sample of 203 deer, 13 per cent were found to be infected (Kingscote, 1950). The snails, *Stagnicola palustris, S. caperata, S. bulimoides, Fossaria modicella, F. parva* and *Pseudosuccinea columella* are reported as intermediate hosts in America. The species exists in Europe also and was in fact first described from deer in a park near Turin. It appears to use here the same snail as the common liver fluke, *Limnaea truncatula,* as its intermediate host, although it also enters *Limnaea peregra* (Erhardová, 1961).

CHAPTER 2

HOSTS OF THE LIVER FLUKE

Mammalian Hosts

THE economic importance of the common liver fluke, of course, lies in the damage it causes to cattle and sheep; but its presence in other mammals is also of interest as it may provide a natural reservoir of infection that would make the elimination of liver fluke disease from a given area more difficult. Furthermore, the range of hosts and the possible differences in the pathological processes in different species are important in the study of host-parasite relationships and specificity.

The rabbit undoubtedly forms a reservoir of infection. Thomas comments that in the 1879–80 outbreak of fascioliasis the wild rabbits of Oxfordshire were decimated and some carried up to 40 or 50 flukes. In Texas, Olsen (1948) examined 309 jack rabbits, *Lepus californicus mezziani,* and 24 cotton tail rabbits, *Sylvilagus floridanus* subsp; 32 per cent of the first and 20·8 per cent of the second were infected.

Other mammals in which the common liver fluke has been found include the deer, kangaroo, wild sheep, dogs, koala, wombat, camel, nutria, mule, horse, donkey, rat, squirrel, beaver, coypus, wild boar; and also, of course, man.

Snail Host

Limnaea truncatula is the acknowledged intermediate host of the liver fluke in Europe; the level of infestation in field samples of this snail has been found to be around 5–6 per cent (Kendall, 1949b). The snail is often difficult to find, its numbers fluctuating enormously from time to time. It also exhibits a polymorphism, as described for example, by Stelfox (1911) for Ireland (Fig. 7).

The difficulty of finding it has apparently led some investigators to state that the species is absent from regions where at some other time it was abundant. Leuckart, for example, was led to suspect *L. truncatula* as the intermediate host by the fact that it was one of the only four snail species occurring in the Faroes. In 1931,

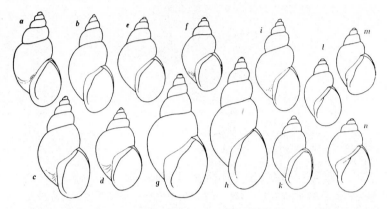

FIG. 7. *Lymnaea truncatula* from different localities. *a*, Stockholm. *b*, Uppland, Sweden. *c*, Gotland, Sweden. *d–e*, Copenhagen. *f, b,* Gentofte, Denmark. *i*, Gottingen. *k,* Sicily. *l, m,* China. (Hubendick, 1951).

Bovien found it abundant on the islands. In 1944, however, Williamson claimed that L. *truncatula* could not be found on the islands although fascioliasis was common in sheep there. Again, the species was generally considered absent from Latvia, until Vaivarina and Viksne (1956) not only found it there but also correlated its distribution to the prevalence of fascioliasis (see also Fig. 8).

Polymorphism as between different populations is widespread not only in *Limnaea truncatula* but also in most other species of the Limnaeidae. Populations of one species may come to resemble those of another species as to size and structure of shell. This may often lead to considerable difficulties in the identification of species, which are discussed by Hubendick (1951). Specimens of L. *truncatula* may be indistinguishable from some specimens of L. *stagnalis*, for example. Hubendick resorts in such cases to the structure of the distal genitalia as a means of species identification. The prostate of L. *truncatula* has one and small inward fold;

L. stagnalis has more than one and unequal folds, some of them ramifying; *L. pereger* and *L. palustris* have one large fold.

From time to time the suggestion is made that other species of snails may also act as the intermediate host. The issue has been investigated in two ways: by sampling natural snail populations for liver fluke larvae, and by attempting the artificial infection of snails of various species with liver fluke miracidia.

Snail hosts outside Europe are listed in Table 2 (see also Fig. 9).

TABLE 2. SNAILS CITED AS INTERMEDIATE HOSTS OF
Fasciola Hepatica OUTSIDE EUROPE

Note: The names of snail species are listed in this Table, and throughout the book, in the form given in the references. The author did not feel qualified to attempt an accurate translation of these to the current nomenclature. It follows that certain different descriptions, for example *Limnaea (Lymnaea) truncatula* and *Glabra truncatula*, refer to one and the same species.

ASIA

Lenia amniata	(Shirai Mitsuji, 1925; Chandraseckariah, 1951) — Japan and India
Limnaea acuminata	(Srivastava, 1944) — India
Limnaea luteola	(Srivastava, 1944) — India
Limnaea allula	(Hagaki, 1958) — Japan
Limnaea pervia	(Kawana, 1940; Ono *et al.,* 1957) — China and Japan
Limnaea philipinensis	(De Jesus, 1935) — Philippines
Limnaea truncatula	is also cited as host in Asia (Kendall, 1956; Watanabe *et al.,* 1955; Srivastava, 1944) or as a new entry (Itagaki, 1958; Japan)

AUSTRALIA AND NEW ZEALAND

Australia	— *Limnaea brazieri; L. launcestonensis; L. subaquatilis.* (References: Ross and McKay, 1929; Johnston and Beckwith, 1946; Smith and Keogh, 1953; Gordon, 1955; Keogh, 1955; Anon., 1956; Gordon *et al.,* 1959).
New Zealand	— Cameron (1951) lists *Limnaea alfredi* and *Mysias ampulla,* while Ross and McKay (1929) incriminate *L. brazieri.* But on reviewing the systematics of Limnaeidae in Australia, Boray and McMichael (1961) conclude that only one species acts as a host of the liver fluke in Australia and New Zealand, and give its correct description as *Lymnaea tomentosa Pfeiffer,* 1855.

(Continued overleaf)

TABLE 2.   SNAILS CITED AS INTERMEDIATE HOSTS OF
Fasciola Hepatica OUTSIDE EUROPE (*continued*)

AFRICA

Limnaea muervensis	(Dinnik and Dinnik, 1956) — Kenya Highlands
Limnaea natalensis	(Fain, 1951; Coyle, 1956) — Congo, Uganda

AMERICA

Limnaea humilis	(McGraw, 1959) — Canada
Limnaea (Fossaria) *bulimoides*	(Shaw and Simms, 1929; Sinitzin, 1929) — North America
Limnaea ferruginea	(Shaw, 1931) — North America
Fossaria modicella	(Krull, 1933a) — North America
Lymnaea traskii	(Krull, 1934) — Florida
Fossaria cubensis	(Van Volkenberg, 1929; Hoffman, 1930) — Florida.
Pseudosuccinea columella	(Krull, 1933d) — Florida
Stagnicola bulimoides *techella*	(Olsen, 1945) — Texas
Limnaea cubensis	(Van Volkenberg, 1929; Hoffman, 1930) — West Indies and South of U.S.A.
Limnaea attenuata	*Limnaea obrussa*; *Limnaea humilis* (Mazzotti, 1955) — Mexico
Limnaea bogotensis	(Muñoz-Rivas, 1953; 1954) — Colombia
Limnaea cubensis	(Ramirez-Villamediana and Vergani, 1949) — Venezuela
Limnaea viatrix	(Tagle, 1944; Faigenbaum *et al.*, 1950; Tagle, 1956)— Argentine and Chile

Population Samples

In an area of Russia where cercaria of the liver fluke could readily be found in L. *truncatula,* Petrochenko (1954) failed to find the larvae in specimens of *Glabra palustris, Radix ovata, R. pereger, Limnaea stagnalis, Physa fontinalis* and *Succinea pfeifferi.* Kastak (1958) had the same experience on examining 68,000 specimens of various fresh-water snails in Czechoslovakia. Again, Mikacič (1960) examined 8369 specimens of L. *truncatula,* 2035 of R*adix pereger* and 268 of *Stagnicola palustris.* Only the first-named species carried the infection, the level of infestation being 4·8 per cent (in March).

L. *pereger* and *Gyraulus hebraicus* were found free of the infection in Turkey (Güralp and Simms, 1959); also, *Glabra palustris, Radix ovata* and *Planorbis planorbis* were free of liver fluke cercaria

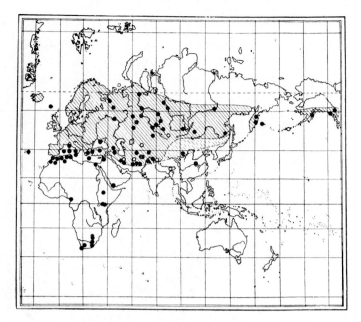

FIG. 8. The distribution of *Limnaea truncatula*. (From Hubendick, 1951).
The hatched lines mark the main area of the species, and the dots mark some of the localities from which records are available.

in areas of Russia where *L. truncatula* did carry the infection (Vasileva, 1960; 964 specimens examined).

The results cited tend to absolve species other than *L. truncatula* of responsibility for fascioliasis in Europe. But Taylor (1922) claimed to have found perfectly developed cercaria of the liver fluke in *Limnaea pereger* in areas in the S.W. of Scotland where fascioliasis is present and *L. truncatula* is rare. In the Leningrad region, Goderdzishvili (1955) failed to find *L. truncatula* but obtained liver fluke cercaria from *Glabra palustris* (5·4%), *Limnaea stagnalis* (1·2%), *Radix ovata* (5·4%) and *Radix pereger* (3·3%).

Laboratory Tests

Thomas and Leuckart, the discoverers of the liver fluke life cycle, themselves resorted to laboratory tests to screen a number of snails that they considered likely hosts.

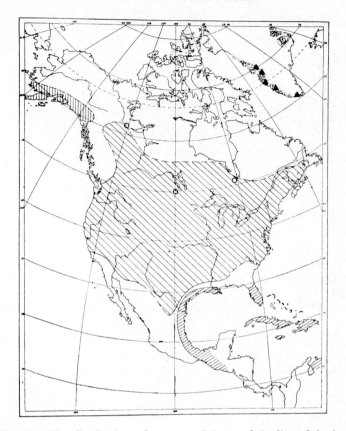

Fig. 9. The distribution of some snail hosts of the liver fluke in North America. (From Hubendick, 1951).
Large ruled area, distribution of *Limnaea humilis*. Small vertically ruled area (in Alaska) and small rings, distribution and localized records of *L. truncatula*. Small transversely ruled area, distribution of *L. cubensis*. Black triangles (in Greenland), distribution of *L. vahli*.

Thomas attempted to infect the following species of snail with liver fluke miracidia — *Limnaea palustris, L. auricularis, L. stagnalis, Physa fontinalis, Planorbis marginalis, Pl. carinatus, Pl. vertex, Pl. spirorbis, Bythinia tentaculata, Paludina vivipara, Succinea amphibia, Limax agrestis, L. cinereus, Arion ater, A. ortensis* and *Limnaea truncatula.* He succeeded only in the case of the last-named species, thus proving that this is the intermediate host he was looking for.

Leuckart on the other hand was misled for a time by his success in infecting *L. pereger,* although he was unable to obtain cercaria from it.

More recently, the contradictory findings from field samples of snails prompted biologists to resort again to controlled laboratory tests.

In one experiment, four out of the six species tested became infected by the miracidia and eventually released normal cercaria capable of infecting mammals. But whilst *L. truncatula* could be infected at any age, the other three species involved (*L. palustris, L. glabra* and *L. stagnalis*) could be infected only when newly hatched. Another two species, *L. pereger* and *L. auricula,* can also be infected but the miracidia fail to develop in them beyond the redia stage (Kendall, 1949a and b, 1950).

In similar tests in Bavaria (Stiegler, 1954), miracidia were found able to penetrate *L. stagnalis* but unable to develop beyond the sporocyst stage; few were able to penetrate into *L. ovata* and again failed to complete development; *Radix pereger* could be entered when newly hatched but not as an adult, and in any case, development in this species stopped at the sporocyst stage; *Stagnicola palustris* was only penetrated superficially, the miracidia failing to proceed beyond the basal connective tissue.

Other species entered by miracidia are: *L. natalensis* and *L. auricularia,* but the infection dies out as the snails become adult (Kendall and Parfitt, 1959).

Goderdzishvili (1955) succeeded in infecting *Glabra palustris, Limnaea stagnalis* and *Radix ovata,* but failed in his efforts to infect *Radix pereger.* However, in field samples he found this latter species infected at a 3·3 per cent level, so that his failure may have been due to the age of the specimens used in the tests. The author does not indicate the stage to which the miracidia were able to develop in the three species entered.

Age of snails was considered carefully by Sazanov (1957). He found both *Glabra truncatula* and *G. palustris* from the Don estuary susceptible when 3–10 days old and *L. stagnalis* throughout the first 30 days of life. The following species could not be infected at any age: *Radix ovata, Planorbis planorbis, Viviparus viviparus,* and *Succinea pfeifferi.*

Bogomolova (1961) found that miracidia penetrated most

specimens of *Limnaea stagnalis, Radix ovata, R. pereger, Galba palustris, G. truncatula* and *Physa fontinalis*; but cercaria were produced only from *G. truncatula* and young *R. ovata*.

The infectivity of snails of one and the same species may vary between populations or for different strains of the parasite. That this may be the case is suggested by some findings of Kendall and Parfitt (1959). Miracidia of *Fasciola gigantica* from Pakistan could infect *Limnaea natalensis* (from Africa) as well as *L. auricularia* (from Pakistan); but South African miracidia, whilst infecting *L. natalensis* easily, could only establish themselves in *L. auricularia* with difficulty.

It may be concluded that miracidia of the liver fluke are undoubtedly able to enter certain species of snails other than *L. truncatula*, particularly if these snails are newly hatched. In only a few species however, probably only *L. palustris, L. glabra* and *L. stagnalis,* do the miracidia develop to cercaria. In others, development stops at some intermediate point.

CHAPTER 3

ENVIRONMENTAL INFLUENCES ON THE LIFE CYCLE

THE complex life cycle of the liver fluke is affected by many environmental conditions, detailed knowledge of which is not only of biological interest but is also relevant to the problem of control of the parasite. Furthermore, environmental factors influence the incidence of liver fluke indirectly, by affecting survival, development and numbers of the snail host (see Chapter 19 and Table 4).

Development of Egg and Hatching of the Miracidium

Temperature
Many tests have shown that the period from the release of the egg to the hatching of the miracidium increases as the temperature decreases (Table 3). Below 5°C, development in the laid egg

TABLE 3. HATCHING PERIODS RECORDED IN VARIOUS TESTS

Temperature (°C)	Hatching period (days)	References
10·5–20°	30+	Ono and Isoda (1951)
11 –19°	45	Tagle (1944)
Room temperature	17–22	Roberts (1950)
25°	8–12	Roberts
21 –26°	17–18	Ono and Isoda (1951)
28 –32°	10–14	Ono and Isoda
25 –31°	9	Tagle (1944)
Warm season in Kenya Highlands	52–70	Dinnik and Dinnik (1959)
Cold season in Kenya Highlands	up to 109	Dinnik and Dinnik

C

TABLE 4. ENVIRONMENTAL CONDITIONS, THEIR EFFECTS ON AND CORRESPONDING ADAPTATIONS OF THE LIVER FLUKE
(FROM STYCZYNSKA-JUREWICZ, 1958)

Environmental conditions	Advantageous effects	Disadvantageous effects	Adaptations of the parasite
Stagnant water		Rotting	Retarded development under anoxic conditions
Running water, floods, permanent streams	Dispersal of eggs and cysts. Dispersal of the snail host. Increased fertility of habitat	Washing away of the miracidia	Cysts boat-shaped and forming at surface of the water
Short rain	Induces emergence of cercaria		Immediate hatching of cercaria
Prolonged rain	Reactivation of dessicated snails		Acceleration of development
Cold		Decreased rate of development and survival	
Frost		Kills eggs and miracidia	
Warm and dry periods		Dries out snail egg masses. High mortality of snails	Fewer larvae in dessicated snails
Warm and wet periods	Accelerated development of eggs and larval stages. Greater activity of snails		Adjustment of development to an optimum temperature corresponding to that of transitory water pools in summer
Numbers of snails	Abundant — Easier infection by miracidia. Larger numbers of cercaria	Scarce — Contact with miracidia less likely. Snails, tend to be old and to live in drier patches	Movements and tropisms of the miracidia
Numbers of mammalian hosts	Abundant — Easier infection with cysts. Fertilization of snail habitat. Hoof-prints as pools of water	Scarce — Contact with snail less likely and less prolonged	Swimming of cercaria. Encystation on grass. Resistance of cysts to adverse conditions
Supply of snail food	Abundant—Large snail populations. Better larval development in well-fed hosts	Scarce — Fewer intermediate hosts, and fewer larvae developing	Production of rediae adjusted to nutritional state of hosts

stops, to be resumed as soon as the temperature returns to 13°C (Krull, 1934). This arrest of development does not seem to apply to the earliest stages. Even when fully formed, the miracidium will not hatch so long as the temperature is too low even for part of the day; it may remain alive inside the egg for up to 105 days, although by the 90th day it has already lost the capacity to develop further. Rowcliffe and Ollerenshaw (1960) stressed the following three conditions necessary for hatching: the eggs must have become freed from the faeces, they must be surrounded by a film of moisture and the temperature must be above 9·5°C; but, above 30°C development is inhibited and at 37°C all eggs die within 24 days (Figs. 10 and 11).

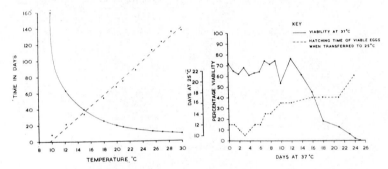

Fig. 10.   Left: effect of temperature on duration of development of the egg; the reciprocal shows speed of development. Right: effect of prolonged incubation of the egg at 37°C and the time which the egg takes to develop when subsequently transferred to 25°C (Rowcliffe and Ollerenshaw, 1960).

The hatching and viability of miracidia have been recently investigated for the species *Fascioloides magna* by Friedl (1960, 1961a) and Campbell (1961b). The eggs can be induced to hatch by a temporary reduction of the partial pressure of oxygen, but good oxygenation is necessary for continued development. Embryonation in this species also occupies about 3 weeks; higher temperatures speed it up but the resulting embryos may be inviable. Storage in distilled water at 5°C does not necessarily kill the eggs. About 50 per cent remained viable after a year, and a few even after two years.

At hatching the operculum of the egg is pushed open. Rowan

(1956) found that it is first loosened by a proteolytic enzyme released by the miracidium under the stimulus of light; this enzyme dissolves the substance binding the operculum to the rest of the shell. The viscous cushion in the egg expands as it comes

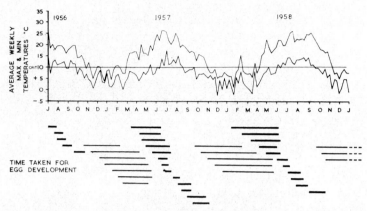

FIG. 11. Relationship between climatic temperature fluctuations and the time taken by liver fluke eggs to develop to the hatching stage outside in the dark (Rowcliffe and Ollerenshaw, 1960).

into contact with water, ruptures the vitelline membrane and flows out of the egg, followed by the miracidium. Incidentally, the enzyme also affects the epithelium of the unhatched miracidium to some extent, causing the loss of salts at that stage.

pH

According to Rowcliffe and Ollerenshaw (1960) the eggs remain viable and hatch between 4·2 and 9·0. Above 8·6 hatching takes three times as long. Mattés (1926) considers the effective hatching stimulus to be a lowering of pH to 5·5–6·0.

Oxygen Content of Water

This factor acts in a complex interrelationship with temperature (Bevejac and Lui, 1959). At 40°C the eggs die in 4 days in oxygen-saturated water, and even a content of 1·9 mg of oxygen per litre of water will inhibit development. On the contrary, at 25°C the embryos remain viable and able to develop in oxygen-saturated water. Reduction of oxygen content delays development and death occurs at levels below 0·2 mg/l. Thus good oxygenation is beneficial at normal temperatures, the optimum being 25–30°C, but becomes detrimental at high temperatures.

The egg cannot withstand drying for more than four days.

Clear water may contain spores of a fungus, *Catenaria anguillulae,* which has been found to parasitise liver fluke eggs. The sporozoa released from the sporangial cysts infiltrate into the interior of the egg, where they give rise to small mycelia on which a new crop of sporangial cysts develops. The fungus can be cultured artificially (Butler and Buckley, 1927; Butler and Humphries, 1932).

Survival of the Free Miracidium

According to Tagle (1944) miracidia live for $5\frac{1}{2}$ hr at 27°C and for 20 hr at 10–13°C, whilst Skvortsov *et al.* (1936) (quoted by Roberts, 1959) found that they remain alive for 40 hr; however, their activity diminishes with time. Villamediana and Vergani (1949) found that miracidia survive for 6–8 hr in water at 30°C and up to 48 hr in a refrigerator.

The minor discrepancies in these various measurements could be due to local differences in liver fluke strains, but also to differences of oxygenation, pH or salinity of the water. For example, the latter authors find that miracidia die within 10 min in saline, and within 8 min in 1 per cent copper sulphate; in weaker solutions of the latter they survive for longer (up to 6 hr in 1:100,000). The presence of lime also kills the miracidia (Gebauer, 1958), even at a concentration of 0·5 per cent.

Penetration into the Snail

For the first few hours after hatching the miracidia keep to the surface layers of the pond water; later they are distributed more evenly and when moribund they sink. They swim in a zig-zag fashion and assume a direction against currents as slow as 1·5 mm/sec (Yasuraoka, 1953).

They are actively attracted to *Limnaea truncatula* mainly, but also to some extent to other species. The chemotactic response is reasonably effective at a distance of 15 cm (Neuhaus, 1953; also Campbell, 1957, for *Fascioloides magna*). The most favourable position for entry is the pulmonary chamber of the snail; but a miracidium will bore even into the foot of the snail (where no further development is possible) and Thomas (1883) described how "in desperation" it will bore or attempt to bore into any object. The snail epithelium is broken down chemically rather than mechanically, probably by external digestion with enzymes from the larva's penetration glands (Dawes, 1960). Boring may continue even through the host liver, or through connective tissue and blood channels to the roof of the body cavity.

In the process of penetration the miracidium sheds its ciliated epithelium, is halved in size and becomes round in shape. Therefore, the larva after its entry into the host is dissimilar from the miracidium and is, more accurately, described as a young sporocyst.

Development in the Snail

Normal Development

Miracidia penetrating into the snail foot degenerate within a day, whilst those entering through softer tissues develop further: for about 3 days (in snails kept at 25°C) they can be found in the preoesophageal region as inert sporocysts, changing subsequently to motile sporocysts; after two further days they become 1 mm *rediae*. By the 14th day the rediae have settled in the digestive gland (or "liver") of the snail and already contain daughter-rediae (the germ balls, from which these arise, can be seen as early as the 8th day). By the 20th day the rediae may contain cercaria or more daughter-rediae. Within a month these fill the snail's hemocoele. Between the 38th–42nd days the shedding of cercaria begins at the rate of a few hundred per day and continues for up to 8 days, followed by the death of the snail (Roberts, 1950). Shaw (1932) observed instances where the snail went on releasing cercaria for over 2 months.

The number of cercaria finally developing from a single miracidium is variable, depending as it does on environmental conditions and nutrition, but can be very large. Injecting snails of the species *Pseudosuccinea columella* with a single miracidium each, Krull (1941) was able to count three months later anything from 14 to 629 cercaria emerging from one snail.

The completion of development within the snail in 41 days was also confirmed by workers in Colombia (Villamediana and Vergani, 1949). However, larval stages may remain and survive for much longer in this host; it has been shown repeatedly that they may pass the winter there (at least if this is mild) and emerge early in the spring, causing the earliest infections of mammals in the new season (Oshanova, 1959 — Sofia region).

Nutritional State of Snail

The nutrition of the snail is of great importance for the development of the fluke larvae. Kendall (1949b) tested this by infecting snails with large numbers of miracidia and keeping some richly supplied with algae and others starved. The first group of 10 well-fed snails grew to 0·82–1·08 cm and yielded in all 14,426 mature cercaria on dissection. The second group of 10 starved snails grew to 0·62–0·64 cm (shell length) and yielded only 2243 mature cercaria. In both cases the snails were dissected 32–41 days after infection. It is noteworthy that the number of rediae was 133–344 per snail in the first group and 30–215 in the second. The number of mature cercaria turned out to be inversely proportional to the number of rediae in the snail. The number of rediae developing from one miracidium is about 40.

Dessication of the snail does not prevent the development of miracidia up to the redia stage, but does not allow the change-over to the production of cercaria; moreover, dessication reduces the viability of infected snails (Styczynska, 1956).

The age of the snail is also important, possibly because of nutritional factors. Development takes twice as long in mature as in young molluscs (Krull, 1934, 1941; on the American snail host *Pseudosuccinella*).

Temperature

In *Limnaea viatrix* in Chile (Tagle, 1944), sporocysts take 9 days to form rediae, and cercaria appear after 37–60 days, depending on temperature. Davtyan (1956) finds that cercaria developing at 22–23°C (in 33–34 days) are more viable and thus are more infective than those developing at 15–17°C (in 64–68 days). At high temperatures of 29–32°C development is speeded up slightly (30–32 days) but the cercaria are less infective than the 21–23° group. Infectivity is a function of viability and absolute numbers. If the temperature falls below 9°C the cercaria fail to emerge from the snail (Kendall and McCullough, 1951).

Development of the Metacercarium

Survival of the Metacercaria

Emergence can be stimulated in the laboratory by transferring the snails to water if they were dry before, or to fresh water if they were in unchanged water for 1–2 days before. Emergence of the cercaria from the perivisceral spaces of the snail is thought to be due to rupture of the mantle cavity wall as a result of activity of the snail. If this is correct the change of water stimulates muscular activity and hence leads to rupture (Kendall and McCullough, 1951).

Grigoryan (1959) studied the survival and infectivity of meta-cercaria under various conditions by infecting sheep with a given number of cysts. Cysts on freshly cut hay kept in the open (temperatures ranging from 21–32°C and relative humidities from 30–50 per cent) were still infective to a 1 per cent level after 15 (but not after 35) days. On lucerne leaves kept in petri dishes in the shade (24–29°C and 60–75 per cent) cercaria remained dangerous for 5 (but not for 15) days. Infective cysts do not survive the process of silage production. If preserved in water, cysts are not infective after 10 months. Over a short period, even with temperatures ranging from −2 to 50°C at least some cysts remain infective. In refrigerator temperature cysts may still be infective after 11 months (Shaw, 1932).

Life-Span of the Adult

The adult stage and the bile duct habitat are reached within about two months after infection with metacercaria. Tagle (1944) obtained adult flukes from rabbits and goats 54 days after infection with encysted cercaria, and Montgomerie (1931) working on rabbits found flukes 10 weeks after infection.

Information as to the life-span of the adult liver fluke is scanty. In some textbooks it has been implied or stated that the flukes leave the host at some time after reaching the adult stage. But Leiper (1938) infected 16 goats which he protected from subsequent reinfection, and 5 yr later he could still obtain fluke eggs from them. Durbin (1952) infected three sheep and took care to exclude accidental infection thereafter. When the animals were slaughtered 8 and 11 yr later they still carried liver flukes. In a similar test, Egorov (1954) infected a 2-year-old sheep and 8 yr later found 22 live flukes in it. Therefore it appears that a liver fluke may live for 8 yr or more.

CHAPTER 4

DISCHARGE OF EGGS FROM THE MAMMALIAN HOST

DETECTION of liver fluke eggs in the faeces of a mammal establishes of course the diagnosis of *fascioliasis*; on the other hand, the absence of eggs does not altogether exclude the presence of parasites, as these may be at the migratory stage that has not yet reached the bile ducts and shed eggs.

The egg of the liver fluke is oval and about 140μ long (Fig. 12). The egg membrane is clear initially but by the time the egg is

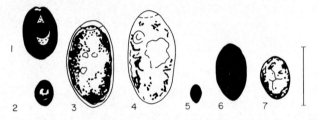

FIG. 12.   Eggs of parasites obtainable from the faeces of mammals by precipitation (redrawn from Borchert, 1954) Vertical line 100μ to scale.

1. *Globidium*   2. *Dicrocoelium*
3. *Fasciola*   4. *Paramphistomum*
5. *Opisthorchis*   6. *Macroconidiorhynchus*
7. *Dipylidium bothrium*

shed it has changed to a thin pale yellow sclerotin cover which still remains transparent. The operculum has a serrated seam.

Most techniques of examination of faecal samples for liver fluke eggs depend on the fact that these, if present, fall to the bottom of the container from a suspension of faecal matter. (Techniques on the principle of floating the eggs are not preferred with this parasite because the eggs are liable to burst in a concentrated solution; although solutions of sodium silicic acid or zinc chloride in saline can be used for flotation procedures.) Nematode eggs also sink, but at a slower rate than the liver-fluke eggs.

On the other hand eggs of paramphistome flukes sink with the same speed as those of the common liver fluke. Dead or malformed eggs of the liver fluke, such as those often appearing after successful medication will float because of gas forming in them.

All variations of the technique comprise in principle, the following steps: the faecal sample is dispersed in water and passed through sieves, usually of 20, 40 and 60 mm to the inch before the final suspension is obtained. In some procedures the suspension is made in beakers or similar vessels, whilst others require special glass tubes up to 2 m high (Someren, 1947; Gregoire et al. 1956).

Sedimentation of the eggs is usually speeded up by the addition of a detergent which loosens them away from other material and from the glass; or a small quantity of 1 per cent aluminium sulphate solution may be used. The precipitate with the eggs is sampled through a tap at the bottom of the tube. To facilitate the observation of the eggs under the microscope, neutral red (or indian ink or carbol fuchsin) is added; this stains most other materials but leaves the eggs as bright colourless spots. Alternatively, tincture of iodine is used, which stains the eggs deep brown. Counts can be made with a haemocytometer or similar device. Carboxymethyl cellulose solution is recommended for an even distribution of eggs within the counting chamber (Dorsman, 1956).

Of course, the amount of faeces, i.e. size of sample, used in the suspension will affect the sensitivity of detection. With samples of 5–6 g Leontiev (1956), found eggs in 10 per cent of 56 cattle; with samples of 20–25 g, 27 per cent of the same cattle were shown to be infected.

In view of the requirements for simplicity, speed, accuracy and standardization of a technique which is often used in the field, many modifications of detail, such as the number of successive dispersions and sedimentations, use of centrifugation or decantation, etc., have been proposed (Van Someren, 1947; Swanson and Hopper, 1950; Stoebbe, 1950; De Jesus and Rivera-Anaya, 1952; Benedek and Nemeseri, 1953; Dennis, Stone and Swanson, 1954; Giamporcaro and Bianco, 1955; Dorsman, 1956; Gregoire et al.,

1956; Teuscher, 1957; Vercruysse and Derde, 1959; Carballeira *et al.,* 1959; Khanbegyan, 1960).

A description of some simple forms that the procedure takes is given in the Appendix.

In addition to their value for diagnosis, repeated egg counts sometimes allow conclusions to be drawn as to the severity of infection and other relevant matters.

Although the uterus of the liver fluke is always full of eggs, the results of faecal counts by Hay (1949) indicate that the maximum rate of release of eggs prevails in the period from March to May, and the minimum in January and February. Even within the same day, there is periodicity, but it is not clear whether this originates in the parasite or is imposed by the host. The hourly rate of egg release rises from morning to mid-day and declines in the afternoon and evening (Dorsman, 1956). It follows that in cases of slight infections there is a better chance of diagnosis by faecal samples taken from the animal's rectum at mid-day.

Can the number of eggs counted give a reliable indication as to the number of liver flukes within the host? Mikacic (1959) investigated this important point, using 100 cattle of different ages and breeds. His results gave an index of

$$\frac{\text{number of adult liver flukes in the host}}{\text{average number of eggs in a 10 g faecal sample}} = 13 \cdot 85.$$

However, this index itself varies with breeds and becomes higher with very severe infections.

Gall Bladder Puncture

As an alternative to examining faeces for fluke eggs, Gomulkin (1957) has described a method for withdrawing bile by puncture of the gall bladder; eggs, if present at all, would be easily detectable in the bile. If properly carried out, the puncture and indeed the application of a plastic tube fistula involves no risk of peritonitis. Gomulkin tested the method on 135 cattle; puncture yielded some bile in 118 of them, whilst in the other 17 the gall bladder was empty. The bile of 60 animals was examined for eggs; 5 animals had eggs of *Dicrocoelium,* and 42 had eggs of *Fasciola* in their bile, although in only 7 of these could liver fluke eggs be found in the faeces. These tests underline the fact that fascioliasis cannot be excluded simply because no eggs of the fluke are found in the faeces.

PART II

STRUCTURE AND PHYSIOLOGY

CHAPTER 5

MORPHOLOGY AND PHYSIOLOGY OF LARVAL STAGES

Embryo

The cleavage of the ovum within the egg, i.e. the series of cell divisions giving rise to the embryo, has been described by Schubman (1905) and by Ortman (1908). The first division gives two unequal cells, a micro- and a macromere. The macromere undergoes two more divisions to give rise to another two micromeres. After this the three micromeres also begin to divide. All the micromeres eventually arrange themselves in a single layer around the macromere, except for one small gap, which may be described as corresponding to a blastopore; and the single macromere may be considered as a single-cell endoderm (Fig. 13). This will give rise to all the endodermal cells. Ortman described the process as "epibolic gastrulation".

Cleavage begins whilst the egg is still in the oviduct, so that by the time it is released from the adult, the egg contains: a cluster of cells near the operculum, the embryo, and a cluster of yolk-cells by its side (Fig. 16). The latter two are surrounded by a clear membrane, produced by the transformation of some cells that are given off by the ectoderm. At least, the histological picture convinced Ortman that the cells making up the membrane around the embryo migrate there from the ectoderm. The yolk-cells have degenerated by this time, but their cell boundaries can still be made out.

Later cell divisions obscure the distinction of two layers; in fact, the morula cells do not fall into differentiated types, and their relative position also seems to be inconstant.

D

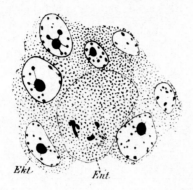

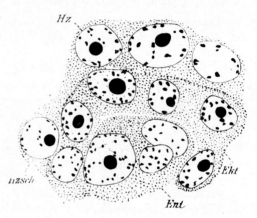

Fig. 13. Sections through early embryos. Top: *Ent,* macromere. *Ect,* micromeres forming the ectoderm. Bottom: At a later stage the endoderm, *Ent,* is made up of the macromere plus products of its divisions. Some cells originating from the ectoderm have moved outwards to form a sheath around the embryo. Between two of these cells, *Hz* and *Hzsch,* there is a gap which has been considered analogous to the blastopore (Ortmann, 1908).

Miracidium

Within 2–3 weeks the miracidium fills the egg. It is equipped with two brown eye spots and performs peristaltic movements.

Within the miracidium, four main cell aggregates become distinct and constitute the primordia of the organs to develop (Figs. 13–17).

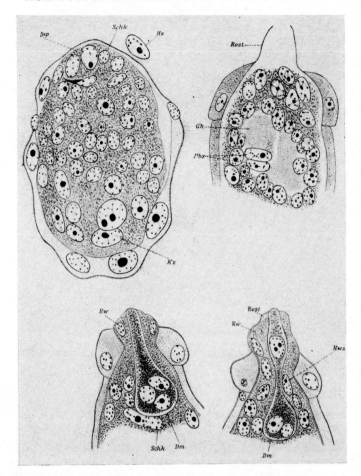

FIG. 14.   Stages in the development of the miracidium. Upper left, larva with the epidermis formed and ciliated. *Dep,* cell from which the gut, *Dm,* develops. *Kz,* germinal cell. *Schk,* shell nucleus. *Rost,* rostellum. *Gh,* brain. *Pbz,* cells forming later the pigmented cup of the ocelli. *Rw,* collar. (Ortmann, 1908).

(a) A group of cells moves to the surface of the embryo, changes shape and coalesces so as to surround the embryo; these cells acquire cilia and become the ciliated epidermis of the miracidium. External examination of the free miracidium will give a clear idea of the structure of its ciliated epithelium. It consists of 21 polygonal cells arranged in five rings of 6, 6, 3, 4 and 2 cells. According to Mattés (1949) these cells are not apposed to each other but there is a ribbon, 2μ wide, between them which

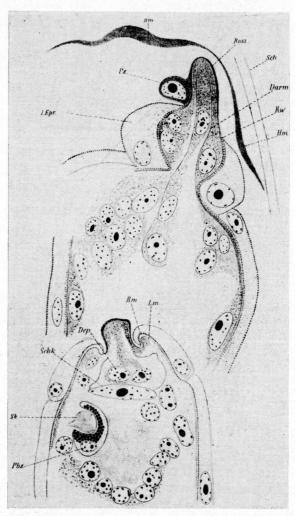

FIG. 15. Further stages in the development of the miracidium. *Rm, Lm,* circular and longitudinal muscle. *Dep,* gut epithelium. *Darm,* gut. *Sch,* egg shell. *Hm,* embryonic sheath. *Pz,* polar cell. Other symbols as in Fig. 14 (Ortmann, 1908).

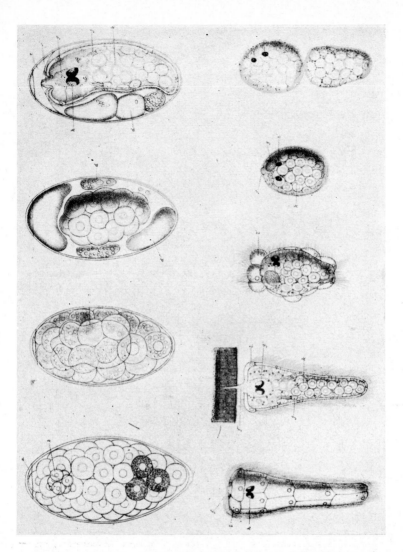

FIG. 16. Stages in the development of the miracidium (Thomas, 1883). Upper left: two figures, early cleavage stages. Upper right: two figures, the formed miracidium within the egg. Lower left: two figures, the hatched miracidium to show its epithelial cells and the mode of penetration into the tissues of the snail. Lower right: three figures, the change of the miracidium into a sporocyst on entry into the snail, and transverse division of a sporocyst. *e*, mucus. *f*, head papilla or rostellum. *g*, rudimentary gut. *j*, ciliated infundibulum. *k*, germinal cell. *i*, ciliated epithelium. *d*, remnants of the yolk. *l*, epaulet cells of the first ectodermal row of cells. *l'*, the disintegrating epaulet cells. *f*, rostellum. *g*, rudimentary gut. *h'*, residual eye spots. The sporocyst may divide transversely as shown in the drawing on the right.

belongs to the body wall underneath. It is on this ribbon that the excretory organs, sensory papillae and side organs open.

The polygonal cells carry cilia in long rows. During penetration into the host these cells become discarded, round off, and can swim as if they were individual ciliates.

Between the first and second rings of epithelial cells are found paired sensory papillae; two dorsal, two central and one lateral pair on each side.

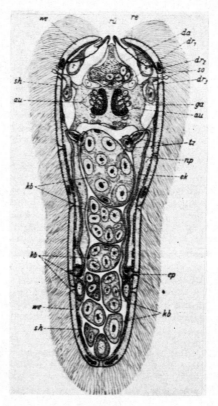

FIG. 17.   Detailed structure of the miracidium.

da, gut. *dr₁,* pharyngeal glands. *dr₂,* anterior mucous glands. *dr₃,* posterior mucous glands. *re,* retractor muscle. *ru,* rostellum. *g,* ganglion. *au,* eye. *sh,* sub-epithelial layer. *tz,* terminal cell of excretory tubule. *np,* nephridial plasma. *ek,* excretory tubule. *ep,* excretory pore. *we,* ciliated epithelium. *Kb,* germ balls (Mattés, 1949).

The body wall under the epithelium is a syncytium, with two layers of muscle fibres: circular and longitudinal from without inwards. The body wall thickens and cell divisions are seen in it after the entry into the snail host.

(b) A group of cells at one pole of the egg enlarge, and their nuclei become vacuolated. These are the primordia of the germ cells.

One of the primordial germ cells forms a sheath around the others. Histochemical tests at the free miracidium stage show that the germ cells have higher nucleic acid and acid-basic protein content than other embryonic cells; in this they resemble the adult reproductive cells (Bogomolova, 1957). In addition, the germ cells are devoid of storage substances such as fat or glycogen.

(c) Some cells give rise to the excretory organs of the miracidium which comprises tubules with a large star-shaped flame-cell at the end (Figs. 36 and 38). The cells responsible have not been identified; Ortman is inclined to think that it is one single cell that gives rise to the excretory canals on each side. Leuckart (1882) assumed that the tubules form from intercellular lacunae, but other workers have considered them as derived from a string of mesodermal cells; Ortman failed to locate either lacunae or a mesodermal string.

(d) The gut primordium comprises four cells with vacuolated nuclei and a fifth with a very small nucleus rich in chromatin, plus a large cell sitting on the rest like a cap. The gut never acquires an opening, nor a lumen, but becomes surrounded by a thin layer of longitudinal muscle; this seems to arise from the last-mentioned large cell. It is interesting that, in Ortman's account, one cell at the anterior end of the gut primordium becomes split off from the animal altogether and thus leaves a gap in the cell covering of the embryo, as if it was to be a mouth. However, the gap does not amount to an opening because the epidermal sheath still covers it. As a matter of fact, the sheath becomes protruded by muscular pressure and forms the rostellum. Workers previous to Ortman did not describe such a detachment of a cell at the tip.

The gut is not used for feeding but is full of a secretion that lyses the snail tissues; in other words the gut is used as a boring gland, as if the lytic process was a case of extracellular digestion.

(e) A cell group situated at the anterior end of the larva gives rise to the "ganglion"; this comprises both a syncytial neural mass of brain and some cells that differentiate to the eye-spots. Each eye-spot comprises a cavity or cup formed by a single pigmented cell, with three spindle-shaped sensory cells fitting in it. There is no lens.

Other cells of the anterior cell-aggregate detach themselves to come between the gut and the ectodermal musculature at the anterior tip of the body, the retractable rostellum. They take positions as the primordia of the retractors of the rostellum and of the head glands. The retractors are thin muscles, obvious only when the rostellum is retracted. The head glands take the shape of a bag filled with some substance staining dark with Heidenheim's haematoxylin, and open to the outside half-way along the rostellum (although Coe described them as opening at the tip of the rostellum).

Mattés (1949) described three pairs of unicellular glands, the existence of which is, however, doubted by Dawes (1960). The 3 pairs described are:

(a) Pharyngeal or salivary; these are difficult to stain, and their secretion is hyaline. They terminate on a point of the pharynx wall which, when the pharynx is protruded, comes to lie at the very tip.

(b) Anterior mucous glands, earlier described as "head glands". These lie in the region of the first epithelial ring and open again into the pharynx. Their secretion is granular, staining blue with azan.

(c) Posterior mucous glands. These are two cells lying closely side by side and open to the body surface between the first and second rings.

Incidentally, it is interesting to note the observation by Soulsby (1957) that sheep serum contains a component which, under certain conditions *in vitro,* kills miracidia; this of course is of no practical importance as the miracidia are not found in the mammalian host. If 0·5 ml of water containing miracidia is mixed with 2 ml of undiluted sheep serum and with complement, the larvae soon lose their mobility, they swell at the anterior end and sink to the bottom of the container within half an hour. This is not an osmotic effect since it does not happen unless guinea-pig complement is present. The complement is inactivated by heating, but the serum component is not affected by heating to 56°C. The effect remains even if the serum is diluted 320 times. It is likely that the phenomenon is associated with particular serum proteins. A somewhat similar phenomenon was observed for the cercaria of certain other species by Culbertson and Talbot (1935).

Sporocyst

As already mentioned, the miracidium on penetration into the snail leaves its ciliated cover behind, and soon assumes a round shape of about half its original volume; it can be described as a young sporocyst (Fig. 18).

In the course of this transformation the miracidium loses by cytolysis its brain ganglion and gut. The eye-spots persist but become detached from each other and lose their typical crescent shape. Up to ten excretory tubules arise by branching of the miracidial tubules (Kawana, 1940) on each side of the body; but it is doubtful whether they open to the surface. They connect to lacunae between the cells of the body wall. Yellow refractile granules partly soluble in acids have been described by Leuckart in the interstices and even in the cells of the tubules.

Occasionally a sporocyst may divide transversely giving rise to two, the one appropriating the head papilla as well as the eye spot.

From a size of 0·15 mm with an elliptical shape, sporocysts may grow in 15 days to 0·5 mm, whilst becoming more sac-like.

Redia

The cavity of this sac becomes filled with clear round cells arising from the germinal cells of the embryo as well as from the epithelial lining of the sac. Soon these become arranged in groups described as morulae or germ balls (Fig. 18).

Each morula flattens on one side; an invagination changes it to a gastrula, which, however, does not have a real archenteric cavity. A spherical pharynx leads to a blind digestive tract with an epithelium of a single-cell layer. Around the pharynx there are

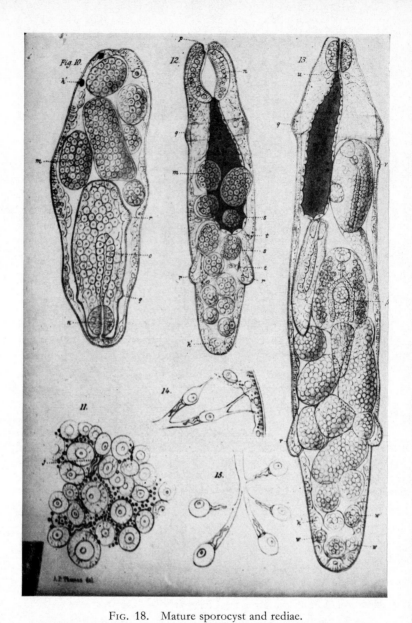

FIG. 18. Mature sporocyst and rediae.

Upper left: mature sporocyst, still carrying the residual eye spot, h'; a redia is forming in it. Upper middle: young redia 0·5 mm long, containing germ balls at different stages of development. The gut is filled with the yellow remains of the snail host's liver tissue. r, posterior processes. t, trabeculae crossing the body wall of the redia. q, collar. w, w', m, s, germinal balls at different stages. k', germ cells. y, cystogenous cells. u, gland cells. B, limbs of the digestive tract of a cercarium forming within the mature redia on the right (Sommer, 1880).

also a few large cells (gland cells) with a duct opening into the junction of gut and pharynx.

The mouth is surrounded by a sphincter muscle and has two folds, or "lips". The pharynx consists of an outside limiting membrane and an inside thick cuticle. The main part of the digestive tract has a single layer wall and a basement membrane; its cells become flattened when the animal distends.

As in the sporocyst, here also there is a definite excretory system embedded in the body wall but it is not clear whether it opens to the outside. The infundibula are branched and there is a flame cell at the tip of each branch. According to Kawana (1940) they are formed by the branching of two tubules already present in the germ ball. Cellular trabeculae or bridges traverse the body cavity from side to side especially at the anterior end. They include fibres and cells with long processes.

Externally, the redia has an annular ridge or collar and two blunt processes like fins. As it approaches a size of 0·26 mm, the redia exhibits active movements and ruptures the sporocyst wall; in some other Trematodes there is a permanent "birth opening". The wound is kept closed by contraction until it heals.

Once the free redia has abandoned the pulmonary cavity and established itself in the liver of the snail host it feeds on the rich tissue and grows 2 or 3 times its initial size. The muscles are now able to contract and distend the body, which does not happen in the sporocyst.

Host Reaction to the Larvae

The pathological changes taking place in snails parasitized by Trematode larvae have been described by Faust (1920), and some further details have been contributed by Agersborg (1924).

The snail "liver" or digestive gland has secretory, absorptive and excretory functions, and consists of racemose tubules (Fig. 19). These all arise from two embryonic out-pockets from the mid-intestine and are lined with glandular epithelium. The tubules are cemented together with interstitial tissue, in which branches of the hepatic artery, blood lacunae, bile ducts, and nerve endings are also to be found. The whole gland is enclosed in a membrane (tunica propia). The palissade cells of the epithelium are irregular in shape, contain a small oval nucleus, and fall into two physiological types: enzyme-secretory cells and absorptive cells. In addition, the epithelium includes rhomboidal or tetragonal lime cells with large spherical nuclei, and numerous granules; according to some authors, the latter contain tri-calcium phosphate.

The miracidia reach the digestive gland from the pulmonary cavity (or other tissues of the snail) through the blood and lymph

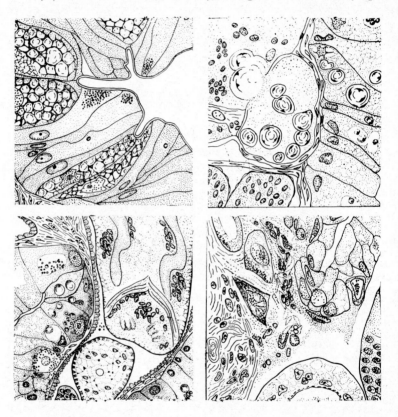

FIG. 19. The damage to the digestive gland of the snail host. Upper left: Cells of tubule of normal liver cell, showing lime cells, liver cells and intertubular connective tissue. Upper right: Cercaria present. Lower left: Cercaria and sporocysts in the connective tissue. Vacuolization of tubule epithelium, from which glycogen is transferred to the parasite. Lower right: Late stage of parasitism with fibrous hypertrophy of the connective tissue (Faust, 1920).

channels rather than through the lumen of the liver tubules; they are always found in connective or interstitial tissue and their first food is lymph.

Lodgement of miracidia (or cercaria) in the tissues give rise to irritation, evidenced by nervous movements of the host. As the miracidia change into sporocysts and grow, the host becomes exhausted and the tubules collapse. The liver does not give positive reactions for fat and glycogen any more, evidence that the parasites have appropriated these nutrients.

Furthermore, waste products of the parasite cause lysis of the cells, alterations of the nuclei and breakdown of cell walls. If the cercaria become encysted in the liver, the interstitial cells hypertrophy and enclose them, in which case the tubular epithelium may recuperate.

Agersborg maintained that the host snail reacts by producing a secretion from the cells of all tissues which is visible as osmium-staining granules in the intercellular spaces; but these granules may in fact be fat droplets released from damaged cells.

Both authors worked with species of snails different from *Limnaea truncatula*, the first with *Planorbis quadelupensis*, *Physoposis africans*, *Planorbis trivolvis* and *Physa sp.*; the second with *Limnaea obrussa*, *Physa gyrina* and *Planorbis trivolvis*. Also, the infections they studied were due to miracidia of various undefined species of Trematodes. However, it is very likely that the histo-pathological picture of the snail liver would not be different in the case of *Fasciola hepatica* in *Limnaea truncatula*.

Cercarium

As noted already, a germinal mass or morula within a redia will develop either to another redia or to a cercarium (Fig. 20). It has been suggested that the "choice" is governed by external conditions; rediae forming in warm weather and cercaria in colder weather. Anyhow, both types of larvae may be found within one and the same redia.

The morula developing in the direction of a cercarium becomes thinner at one end to form a tail, whilst the oral and ventral suckers take shape at the other end. A pharynx, oesophagus and two-limbed intestine constitute a blind and in fact solid alimentary system, although it does acquire a fine lumen later. It has no feeding function however.

Cell inclusions and secretions have been described. Two groups of cells, situated on the ventral side contain cystogenous

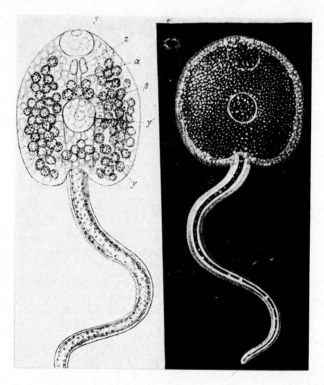

FIG. 20.   Structure of the cercarium.
y, oral sucker. *z*, pharynx. *α*, oesophagus. *β*, limb of digestive tract.
y′, ventral sucker. *y*, cystogenous cells; against a dark background
(middle) these appear opaque (from Thomas, 1833).

refractive granules. The two groups later coalesce and their contents make the cercarium opaque.

Rod-shaped granules are contained in other large, parenchymatous cells situated on the dorsal side. The rods have been variously described as spines or muscle fibrils or even as bacteria.

These cells are probably identical with the "pin cells" described by Braun (Brönn's Thierreich, 1879–1893).

In the sub-cuticle of the dorsal and lateral sides and along the tail of the cercarium Krudenier (1953) found mucoid gland cells.

The excretory system develops in the cercarium by the branching of two tubules forming in the germ ball (Kawana, 1940) and may be described by reference to the diagram given by Rees (1932) (Fig. 21).

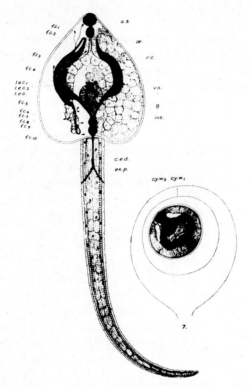

Fig. 21. Structure of the cercarium, to illustrate especially the excretory system. Explanation of symbols in the text (Rees, 1932).

The excretory vesicle is bi-lobed. One duct emerges on each side and proceeds forward to the level of the pharynx; it then returns backward and up to the ventral sucker, then it follows the intestine and further on it loops forwards again. The first part of the duct, from vesicle to loop, is very wide and filled with excretory granules. Ten flame cells at tubule terminations are found on each side; Wright (1927) could only count 7 of them.

The vesicle or excretory bladder is formed, as in all cercaria (La Rue, 1957), by the confluence of the caudal parts of the two excretory tubes. In the Fasciolidae the bladder is originally thin-walled but later becomes overlaid with muscle fibres and other elements.

The excretory system does not extend to the tail, except for a central caudal duct for the first 1/5 only of tail length. As the cercarium matures the caudal parts of the excretory vessels regress and a new pore forms at the junction of body and tail. There is no agreement as to the origin of the cercarian excretory system (see discussion of the system in the miracidium).

As the cercarium, although free-moving, does not feed it must contain stores of energy-yielding substances. In a histochemical examination of cercaria of various species, Ginetsinskaya (1960) detected glycogen granules in the suckers, the walls of excretory tubules and the parenchyma. She could also follow the dis-appearance of the carbohydrate and found that it occurs earlier at higher temperatures. Compared to other species, liver fluke cercaria are not particularly rich in glycogen.

Polyembryony

It has been argued in the past that the "germinal balls" or "germinal masses" in the sporocysts and rediae are formed by the division of ova produced by these same larval stages. Sporocysts and rediae would in that case be neotenous forms producing haploid ova, and these would develop parthenogenetically. This theory of "heterogeny" has now been set aside; the germinal masses are thought to consist of somatic cells from the original zygote. Whilst other contemporary cells are differentiating to produce the tissues of the following larval stage, these germinal ones remain embryonic and inert and are available for the differentiation of the subsequent larval stage; then again some of their number would remain unused to constitute further germinal masses.

When some of the cells of a germinal mass start dividing and differentiating into a multicellular incipient embryo of the next larval stage, the mass will comprise both germinal cells and such multicellular bodies. The latter will eventually detach themselves to form the new generation of sporocysts or rediae.

This theory of "polyembryony of the original zygote" is discussed by Cort *et al.* (1948) who have described the process in many Trematodes of the order Echinostomidae, though not in *Fasciola* itself.

Cyst and Development to the Adult Stage

On emergence the cercarium swims for a while until it becomes attached to grass. It then assumes a spherical form, mucus flows over its surface and the tail is pinched away within 12 min. The detached tail can maintain its movement for another 6 min. The larva is now called metacercarium and is surrounded by a two-layered protective cyst.

It is in this state that the cyst reaches the stomach of the grazing sheep, cow or other final host. Excystation is mediated by the action of host enzymes; it can be followed *in vitro* as described by Wikerhauser (1960). If metacercaria are placed in a saline solution and transferred to an incubator excystation will not occur. A succession of enzyme solutions is required, namely, pepsin followed by trypsin, i.e. the same sequence of enzymes as that met with in the host's digestive tract (Fig. 22, and see p. 192).

The indispensability of digestive enzymes for the excystment of metacercaria is doubted by Dawes (1961), because he recovered larvae from cysts injected into the peritoneal cavity of mice. Furthermore he found directly that excystment may occur in the digestive tract of species quite unrelated to the natural hosts, namely birds. Not only did excystment take place but there was also some growth of the flukes in the abdominal cavity.

Maturation of the Metacercarium

It is obvious that physiological and metabolic studies cannot make much progress unless a suitable medium becomes available for the maintenance of the parasite *in vitro*. However, such studies — and in fact the assessment of various media — depend also on a detailed knowledge of growth and differentiation of organs and functions. Thus, although some media may maintain

E

life for a period, they may not allow normal development of the organism and may either delay or frustrate it altogether. The signs of normal development for a species are set out usually in the form of "Normal Tables", which are very useful works of reference for research workers.

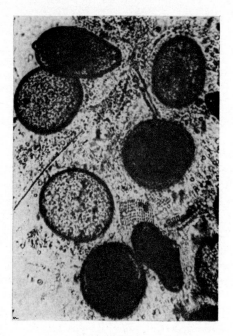

FIG. 22. Excysted metacercaria among cysts, two of them empty. The outer layer of all cysts was experimentally digested *in vitro* with pepsin (Wikerhauser, 1960).

This task was recently accomplished for the liver fluke by Dawes (1962b). He described the growth and differentiation from metacercarium to adult stage on the basis of about 400 specimens recovered from experimentally infected mice. It is interesting that the liver fluke grows faster in the mouse than in its larger natural hosts, reaching maturity and releasing eggs within 5–6 weeks, as against 10–14 weeks in sheep (Montgomerie, 1928). Therefore the timetable of development will be different in the ruminant, but the succession of stages will be as described in the mouse.

These successive stages are shown in Figs. 23–25 from Dawes's paper and are only briefly described here, as the original work should be consulted for its wealth of detail and excellent photographic illustrations.

1. *Metacercarium.* As obtained from cysts recovered from the host, the metacercarium is smaller in size than the cercarium, due to loss of material during the copious secretion of the cystogenous glands. The oral sucker is not quite terminal yet, and the ventral sucker still lies near the posterior end. The gut bifurcates round the ventral sucker but each branch is itself simple, and has a narrow lumen with the gut epithelium cells forming large "beads" along it. Two cell aggregates or organ rudiments are obvious: one in the oesophageal area, from which the cone will grow; another extending medially from the ventral sucker backwards as a coiled structure and destined to give rise to the genital complex and gonads (Fig. 23).

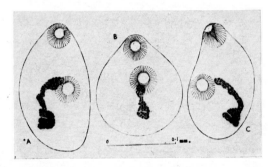

Fig. 23. Flukes recovered from a mouse about 22 hr after infection (Dawes, 1962a). The oral and ventral suckers and the genital rudiment are shown.

3rd day. Flukes recovered three days after infection of the host are larger, and are oval in outline. The gut caeca begin to appear and the genital rudiment is somewhat enlarged, in comparison with the previous stage (Fig. 24A).

8th day. Size is about double that of the metacercarium. The lateral outgrowths of the gut are club-shaped at the end (where they will later bifurcate). The two testis rudiments are now separated from the posterior end of the genital aggregate as two irregularly shaped balls, arranged one behind the other (Fig. 24B).

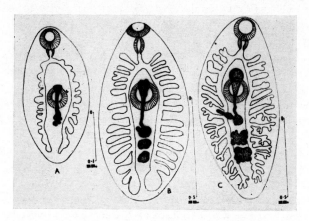

Fig. 24. Flukes recovered three days A, eight days B, and eleven days C, after the experimental infection of a mouse (Dawes, 1962a).
Note the progressive subdivision of the intestinal caeca, and the separation of the testes and ovary rudiments from the initially single genital rudiment.

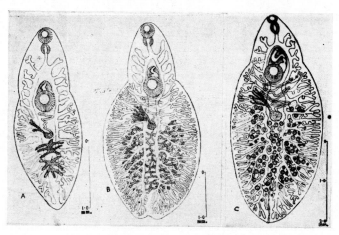

Fig. 25. Flukes recovered from the experimental host fifteen days A, twenty-one days B, and twenty-eight days C, after infection (Dawes, 1962a).

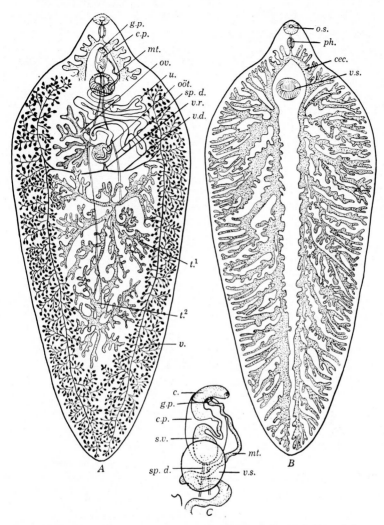

FIG. 26.   Drawings to show the main organs of the adult liver fluke (from Chandler and Read, *Introduction to Parasitology,* Wiley and Sons, 10th ed., 1955).

A. Reproductive system.   Male system; t_1, t_2 the two branched testes *sp.d.,* the sperm duct from the testis to the cirrus. The cirrus, *c,* can be retracted in the cirrus pouch, details of which are shown in C. The sperm ducts, one from each testis, open into a seminal vesicle, *s.v.* from which the cirrus itself begins (see also Fig. 43).   (*cont. on p.* 62)

11th day. The anterior cone is clearly demarcated and contains the four most anterior gut caeca. Behind the ventral sucker, the gut caeca now have secondary and tertiary branches. The rudiment of the ovary is budding off from the main genital rudiment (Fig. 24C).

15th day. The four anterior caeca bifurcate at their terminations. The rudiment of the cirrus is well marked and the testes have developed branches. The shell gland, still incompletely formed, stains deeper than other organs and is thus obvious at the centre of the body. Posterior end of the body still pointed (Fig. 25).

21st day. Posterior end of body now becomes rounded at the tip. The testes are approaching the follicular stage but the ovary is still at the stage of initial branching (Fig. 25).

28th *day.* Fluke already in the bile ducts or about to reach them. Testes now follicular (Fig. 25).

Mature stage (37th day or earlier). Vitelline follicles mature. Egg production.

Whilst it is to Dawes that we owe the thorough description of developmental changes and of the pattern of growth of the adult fluke in the course of its maturation in the mammalian host, some relevant observations had been recorded much earlier by Joseph (1883) and mainly by Bugge (1927a). The first author, in the same year that the elucidation of the life history of the parasite became known, recognized its cysts in the gut, and the early adult stages (with unbranched gut) in the liver and suggested a connection between the two. The second author arranged by size a large number of flukes recovered from mesenteric lymph nodes and livers of affected sheep and cattle. He described how in the smallest (·24 mm long) the gut shows only the primary diverticula

---

Female system: *ov,* single branching ovary leading to the ootype, *oot.* The coiled uterus *u* follows and distally enters the cirrus pouch, where it differentiates into a portion with glandular walls, the metraterm, *mt.* It opens to the outside at the atrium, next to the cirrus (see also Figs. 43 and 48).

B. The bifurcating, branching gut. Note that there is no anus. *o.s.,* oral sucker on which the gut opens. *ph,* pharynx. *cec,* caeca. *v.s.* ventral sucker; this does not connect in any way with the gut but is shown in the diagram as a point of reference.

or caeca (generally twelve in number) and the bladder is situated ventrally, whilst in the mature phase it comes to lie dorsally. He also observed that growth takes place mainly in the part behind the ventral sucker, and that the reproductive glands appear first when the fluke has reached about 1·6 mm.

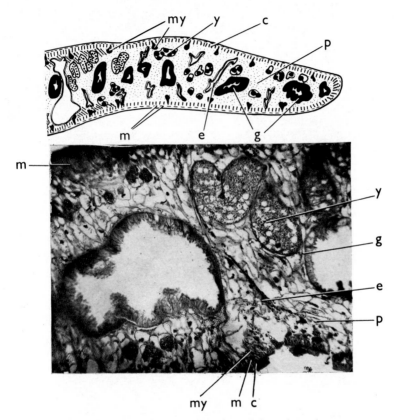

FIG. 27.   Part of a transverse section of an adult to show the arrangement of the main tissue elements and explanatory diagram.

c, cuticular epithelium. *m*, muscular layers. *my,* myoblasts. *p,* parenchyma. *g,* gut with its single-cell epithelial layer. *y,* yolk glands. *e,* excretory tubules containing fat droplets stained black by fixation in Flemming's solution (original).

(The general arrangement of the main systems in the adult, and the high degree of branching of the vitelline, genital and digestive organs are shown in Fig. 26. The position of organs and tissues is shown diagrammatically and in a microphotograph of a transverse section in Fig. 27.)

CHAPTER 6

TEGUMENT AND MUSCLE LAYERS

Cuticular Epithelium

The surface of adult trematodes is covered by a "cuticle", the origin and nature of which has for long baffled investigators. No nuclei or cellular structure could be discerned in it and the description "cuticle" implied an analogy to the chitin of Arthropods.

Concerning the origin of this layer, some favoured the idea that it is the degenerate remnant of an epidermis, or the basement membrane of an epidermis subsequently lost. Others believed that the cells producing the cuticle were retained, and were actually the ordinary mesenchymal cells or, alternatively, epidermal cells which have "sunk" into the mesenchyme.

The problem is important from the phylogenetic point of view, and also from the physiological point of view, as the "cuticle" provides a large area of contact — and possibly of metabolic exchanges — between host and parasite. The nature and structure of this layer has been studied by histological and histochemical techniques, and more recently by electron microscopy.

Alvarado (1951) has, in an exhaustive paper, discussed the various theories critically and has studied the problem by histological techniques. He used the silver-tannin staining techniques of Achúcarro and of Rio Hortega, and the silver carbonate technique of Rio Hortega. By these methods he could differentiate the following layers (Fig. 28): (a) a basal connective membrane, (b) a limiting or hyaline membrane, (c) a cuticular epithelium, and (d) a true surface cuticle. Of these layers, the cuticular epithelium is the thickest and most complex. In addition to the spines, it contains vertical, parallel, tapering tonofibrils, cemented together by a cytoplasmic reticulum. Between the tonofibrils, chains of radially arranged granules (described as chondrioma) can be seen.

The tonofibrils do not reach the basement membrane, but fine extensions from this membrane appear intercalated with them; this, however, does not prevent the easy "peeling off" of the basement membrane from the body which often occurs in fixed specimens. The spines are also in fact bunches of tonofibrils, pressed together.

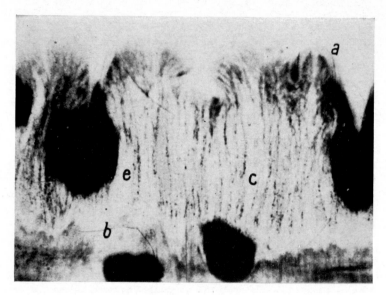

FIG. 28.   The cuticular epithelium in transverse section stained by the silver carbonate method.
c, cytoplasm with rows of mitochondria. *a*, cuticle. *e*, spine. *b*, basal membrane weakly stained (Alvarado, 1951).

The surface cuticle does not stain with Achúcarro's technique or with carbonate pyridine. However, short vertical rods are seen in it; they may represent pores filled with some material which stains with haematoxylin.

Alvarado furthermore felt confident that cell nuclei could be seen in the "cuticle", albeit scarce and in various stages of degeneration. On this basis, the cuticle should be a cellular epithelium, the fibrils and the cytoplasmic reticulum representing differentiated parts of the cytoplasm.

Rather different conclusions were reached by Threadgold

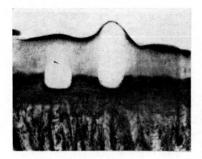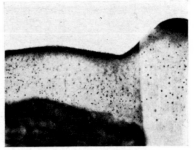

FIG. 29. Left: Part of a section of the "cuticle" of the adult liver fluke, showing a PAS-positive rim and glycogen granules. Part of the spine to the right. Right: Similar section after 3 hr treatment with amylase (Björkman *et al.*, 1963).

(1963a and b) who examined the cuticle and adjacent cell layers under the electron microscope. The cuticle appears as a layer of protoplasm separated from the nucleated main body of the corresponding cells but still connected to them by cytoplasmic strands. These cells are to be found in the cell clusters described in the past as either "glands" or "myoblasts" (see below). The "cuticle" therefore is no inert layer or a secretory product of cells; it does in fact contain mitochondria and membranes of endoplasmic reticulum. The fibrils described by Alvarado are resolved into columns of cytoplasm with chains of mitochondria, and the "nuclei" into irregular masses of mitochondria (Fig. 28). Prenant (1938) has stated the objection to a theory of "insunk ectoderm": no cells in the process of actually "sinking in" have been described. In his view the myoblasts coexist in the cercarium with the true epidermis. A study of immature stages of the liver fluke might provide the answer.

Whether described as a cuticle or as a cytoplasmic tegument, the body covering is much differentiated into successive layers, and some information about their nature has been obtained by histochemical studies, the most thorough being that of Monné (1959). He finds that the basal membrane stains like connective tissue, in fact it gives several reactions similar to the mammalian collagen (blue with Azan, intense colour with Tanzer-Unna, reduces silver nitrate). It is positive to PAS — therefore a polysaccharide —

and remains so after treatment with saliva, hence it is not glycogen (Fig. 29). The spines seem to contain no polysaccharides, nor do they contain polyphenols (unlike the basal membrane). They must therefore be composed of an untanned protein, resembling keratin.

The cuticular epithelium itself, or main cuticular layer of Monné, contains the radial rows of granules (Alvarado's "chondrioma") which give reactions of non-glycogen, probably non-acid, polysaccharides. The fibrils stain with azan blue, like collagen. As to the external membrane or true surface cuticle, it gives the reactions of a protein, with no polysaccharide, and is tanned with polyphenolquinone. Berthier (1954) and Lal and Shrivastava (1960) also obtained positive reactions for muco- or glycoprotein in the cuticle.

The coagula often found on the surface of the worm are definitely acid mucopolysaccharides. The inference is that granules of polysaccharide are excreted onto the surface through the pores of the cuticular epithelium and become acid once on the surface. They may have a protective function against host enzymes.

Björkman et al. (1963) have subjected the surface of adult liver flukes to the action of a battery of enzymes, with the results shown in Table 5. These confirm the predominantly proteinaceous nature of the tegument.

Yamao and Saito (1952) detected phosphatases in the cuticle.

Muscle

The muscles below the cuticular epithelium are arranged in two layers (Fig. 31). Uppermost is the transverse followed by the longitudinal layer. In addition, there is a diagonal layer, but this is restricted to a zone along the dorsal and ventral midlines of the body. Despite some claims to the contrary, no muscles attach to the spines.

Another layer of muscle fibres, crossed in all directions, surrounds the gut. Alvarado commented that because of this arrangement, the muscles cannot push the gut contents in one direction, but can only constrict or dilate the crura (see p. 75).

Dorsoventral muscle fibres are particularly abundant near the

TABLE 5. EFFECT OF ENZYMES ON THE CUTICLE OF LIVE LIVER FLUKES

Enzyme	Activator	pH optimum	Effect
Proteolytic enzymes			
Trypsin Worthington cryst 1961		7·0	—
Papain, Pharm.		4·0–8·1	+
Ficin, Worthington 1961		4·0–8·5	+
Aspergillus oryzae protease, cryst			
(T. Astrup)		6·0–7·0	+
Pronase, Calif. Corp.			
Brochen Res. 1961		7·0	+
Carbohydrate splitting enzymes	NaCl	4·5–7·0	—
α — Amylase, Saliva purified		4·5–7·0	—
α — Amylase, Zymola, DDS		4·5–5·5	—
Lysozyme, Worthington 1961		4·5–7·0	—
Hyaluronidase, Worthington 1961		4·5–7·0	—
Lipolytic enzymes			
Lipase, Worthington 1961	Ca^{++}	6·0–7·6	—
Phospholipase C, 1961		5·1–5·9	—
Phospholipase D. Calif. Corp.			
Brochen Res. 1961			—
Enzyme mixture			
Helix pomatia hepato-pancreas			
homogenate			—

(+ indicates disintegration of the cuticle within 3 hr from immersion in a solution of 0·01 g of enzyme in 3 ml 0·15 M NaCl) (from Björkman *et al.,* 1963).

edges of the worm. Some do not proceed from dorsal to ventral surface but diverge half-way to link with the peri-intestinal muscle layers. Terminally, they insert between the diagonal and longitudinal muscle fibres; occasionally, they reach even into the transverse layer but cannot be seen to attach to the basement membrane. All muscles are invested, like certain other tissues, in a network of fine reticulin fibres (Fig. 41).

The fibres making up the peripheral muscle layers lack nuclei. They have to be viewed therefore as products or parts of cells

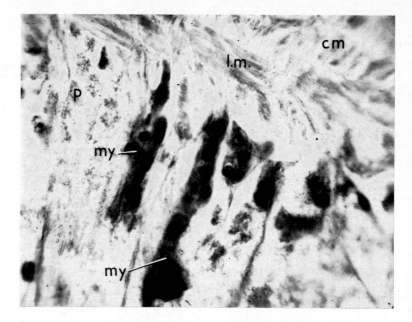

Fig. 30. Detail from a transverse section of an adult liver fluke showing some groups of deeply staining "myoblast clusters" under the muscle layers. *my*, myoblasts. *cm*, circular muscle. *lm*, longitudinal muscle. *p*, parenchymatic cells.

rather than as whole differentiated cells. It was not clear until recently where the nucleated cell bodies were to be found.

Fig. 31. (*opposite*) Diagram to show the relationship of the peripheral tissues in the adult liver fluke as revealed by the electron microscope (L. T. Threadgold, original).

mi, rows of mitochondria in the tegument; also mitochondria in the cytoplasm of parenchymatic and cluster cells. *sp*, spines. *cm*, circular muscle, *lm*, longitudinal muscle, *ep*, epithelial cell communicating by protoplasmic strands to the surface cytoplasmic layer formerly considered as a cuticle. *my*, muscle cells with strands enclosing parts of the cytoplasm differentiated into the muscle fibres.

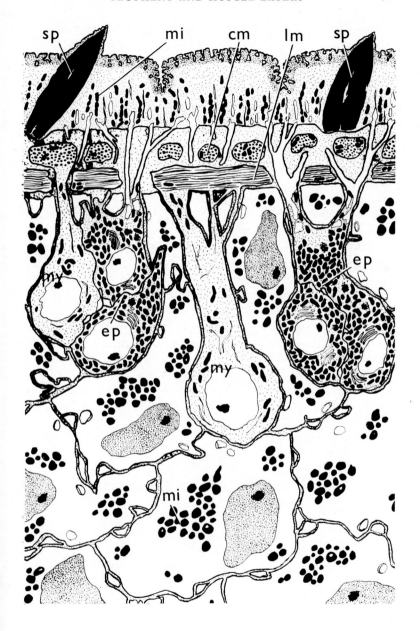

Myoblasts, Gland Cells or Epithelial Cells ?

Below the peripheral muscle layers there are at intervals clusters of cells distinct from the neighbouring parenchyma. Cell boundaries are indistinct and each cluster is probably a syncytium. Logachev (1961) stated that in younger flukes the clusters are fewer and contain fewer nuclei. Hein (1904) who studied these cells mainly in *Distomum lanceolatum*, and to a lesser extent in the liver fluke, claimed that their cytoplasmic extensions traverse the muscle layers, end in spherical "knobs" and are actually apposed to the cuticle. According to his interpretation, these are epithelial cells which, after giving rise to the acellular "cuticle", have sunk deep into the tissues. Bettendorf (1897) also spoke of "large cells" sending "pseudopodia" to the muscle layers.

Others have described these cells as glands, Brandés (1892) being perhaps the first to express this view. Alvarado attributed to these cells the role of muscle cells or myoblasts, mainly on the grounds that each cluster and its neighbouring muscle fibres are all wrapped up in the same network of reticulin. Moreover, he observed that in one particular organ, the cirrus, these myoblasts fill the whole tissue. Their arrangement in clusters elsewhere may be attributed to compression by the vesiculate cells of the parenchyma. The gut muscles have their own myoblasts.

The way in which this controversy has been resolved by a new technique, i.e. electron microscopy, is interesting. It has been noted already that Threadgold (1963) detected strands of protoplasm connecting some of the cells in these clusters to the surface cover of the body. In addition he has found that other cells of the clusters have extensions which enclose the fibres of the muscle layers (Fig. 31). Some of these cells are therefore myoblasts whilst others function as epithelial cells.

CHAPTER 7

FEEDING AND GUT

Food of the Parasite

Early workers, including Leuckart and Sommer (1880), believed that the liver fluke feeds on blood. Evidence for this idea was provided by the presence in the parasite's intestine of iron (Weinland and Brand, 1926) and even of whole blood cells ('Hsu, 1939, cited by van Grembergen, 1950).

Müller (1923) disagreed on the grounds that he could not detect crystals of hemin in the parasite's gut. He suggested that the worm feeds on bile and protein found in the bile ducts. Macé in 1881 (quoted by Braun, 1879–93) had claimed the presence of bile salts in the gut, but others (Küchenmeister, quoted by Macé; and later, van Grembergen) failed to detect any bile acids.

The question of bile in the fluke's intestine was taken up again by Stephenson (1947). For his histochemical tests he fixed segments of bile ducts with the contained worms. He demonstrated that the outer layer of the ducts contain collagen and yet no collagen could be found in the parasites. The inner layers of the bile duct walls contain glycogen (in the racemose glands) but this also could not be found in the parasite. He then proceeded to identify histochemically the brown material usually found filling the lumen of the parasite's gut. From tests with a combination of solvents and bleaching agents he concluded that it is a "malarial pigment", i.e. haematin; it does indeed give the corresponding absorption spectrum at 650λ. Because of the density of pigment in the gut (the corresponding volume of blood being six times that of the pigment), Stephenson was led to believe that the main food of the parasite is blood.

In vitro, adult liver flukes do ingest blood from a blood clot in saline, and the blood ingested can be followed to the crura of the gut, where its colour changes to bluish red. The concentration of

F

this pigment increases for about 3 hr whilst part of it changes to brown granular pigment behaving like acid haematin. No further visible changes occur until defaecation, 24 hr later. The scheme arising from these observations is: blood ⟶ oxyhaemoglobin reduced to haemoglobin ⟶ concentration ⟶ haemolysis ⟶ acid haematin. To this, van Grembergen (1950) added another step: from haemoglobin Fe^{++} to methaemoglobin Fe^{+++}. In fact, the gut contents did not give him a Fe^{++} positive reaction, but a Fe^{+++} positive; with sodium thiosulphate, the contents

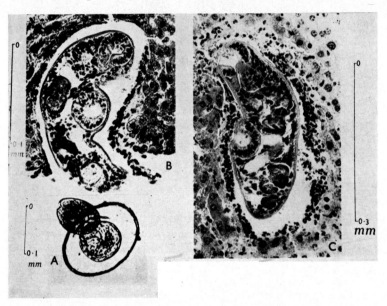

FIG. 32. B and C — Sections of parasitized liver including longitudinal sections of young flukes at the migratory stage. The way in which the parasite feeds on liver tissue can be seen clearly. A. — metacercarium in the process of excystation (Dawes, 1961a).

recreate the haemoglobin absorption band (which haematin cannot do), hence the presence of methaemoglobin was deduced.

Further, Schumacher (1938) and Dawes (1961) have shown histologically by infecting mice with metacercarial cysts that the young flukes burrow their way through the liver for a week or more and in the meantime grow to four times their initial size, so that they are undoubtedly feeding on liver tissue (Fig. 32). Although they must of course ingest some blood, they appear if anything, to avoid blood vessels and to be concerned with the liver tissue itself.

However, a paradox still remains in connexion with the adult flukes that crowd the bile ducts. Do they return to the liver or at least to finer bile ducts for feeding (such feeding migrations to small bile ducts have been suggested by Weinland and Brand, 1926), or do they require no further food? Do they now obtain any nutrients from the bile? The fact that they are found in thick compact clusters makes it improbable that they are able to move to and from the liver tissue or that they can have access to any useful material in the bile, but direct evidence is still wanting on this point.

It may be a relevant fact that *in vitro* the rate of respiration (measured in Warburg's respirometers) of some other parasites (*Hymenolepis* of the rat, *Oochoristica* of the mouse) is inhibited by bile salts (Rothman, 1958).

The faeces are shed through the only opening to the gut, that in the oral sucker. By contractions of the walls of the gut crura the gut contents are moved into the main intestinal branches. From there they are further pushed on towards the anterior end by the contractions of the whole body and the cephalic cone. It takes about 24 hr for material to be thus disgorged, and it is probable that some useful nutrients are also rejected and wasted. Disgorgement does not take place if the cephalic cone is cut; then, despite the continued contractions of the rest of the body, the faeces stay in the gut (Rohrbacher, 1957).

The Gut Epithelium

The gut epithelium is made up of a single layer of cells; some of these are tall and others short, and they carry abundant long fine loops (Fig. 33) on their free edge. Now, the gut epithelium must be responsible not only for absorption but also for some secretion of enzymes, because digestion is undoubtedly (at least partly) extracellular, as shown by the breakdown of haemoglobin in the gut lumen. The question arises which are the absorptive

and which the secreting cells, or does each cell perform both functions, simultaneously or in phases? As he was unable to detect
any histological differentiation, Müller (1923) concluded that all
cells are both absorptive and secretory in function, and that they
become flat and short after discharging their secretion; however,
Stephenson estimated that both high and short cells have about
equal volumes; he did agree with Müller on the dual function of
the cells but could not correlate it with certainty to any gross
changes in cell form.

Gresson and Threadgold (1959) found that the cells are flat in
sections of the gut distended by food and tall in empty areas.
Further, they drew attention to some of the tall cells with a curved
outward side apparently containing a large apical drop of material
(Fig. 33). Their interpretation is that the secretory cells lack
processes but rapidly become transformed to the absorptive phase
with processes; or, alternatively, that some cells are absorptive
throughout but change shape and size depending on the presence
of food. The absorptive processes appear tubular in electron
micrographs.

More recently, Dawes (1962) has thoroughly re-investigated
the whole problem of the gut epithelium by histological methods.
He agreed that the short cells are cells in the absorptive phase, and
provided evidence to the effect that the tall cells are in a stage of
preparation of secretion; this accumulates in apical vacuoles. As
soon as food arrives in the crura the vacuoles of secretion at the
apex of the gut cells in these crura burst and empty into the gut
lumen; but it takes some time before all the residual secretion is
liberated from the cells. The long processes of the cells are
interpreted as due to the breakage of cell walls, associated with
this apocrine mode of secretion.

Again from the study of histological sections, Logachev (1960)
believes that some of the cells of the gut epithelium actually
migrate into the mesenchyme, where they lyse and produce an
intercellular fluid.

The loss of blood in fascioliasis was re-investigated by Pearson
(1963), again with the use of radioactive chromium as a tag for
red cells. Two hours after the injection into the animals used
(guinea pigs and sheep) of tagged red cells, flukes collected from
the main bile duct carried an amount of radioactivity equivalent

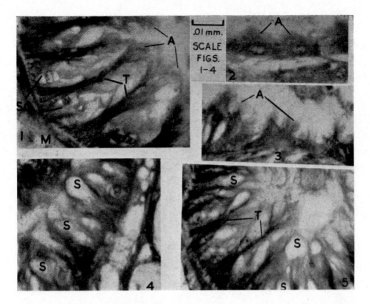

Fig. 33. Transverse sections of part of the intestinal epithelium. *M,* muscle surrounding the gut. *S.C.,* short cells, interpreted as in an early phase of secretory cycle. *T,* tall cells with the protoplasmic (interpreted as absorptive) processes, A. *S,* secretion contained in the free ends of gut cells (Gresson and Threadgold, 1959).

to 0·26 ml of 0·015 ml of blood, or 0·180 ml per day per fluke. This figure agrees well with that of 0·2 ml from the work of Urquhart *et al.* on rabbits. At the same time, each ml of bile from the main duct carried an amount of radioactivity corresponding to 0·26 ml of blood. It is therefore possible, that the chromium is absorbed by the flukes in the duct from the bile itself, rather than directly from blood on which they feed. In other words, it cannot be decided on this evidence whether the flukes in the bile duct feed on blood or not. However, the bile of a non-infected control sheep had only the activity corresponding to 0·01 ml of blood/ml bile. But the release of chromium into the bile of the infected animals might be attributed to the less mature flukes living in the smaller bile ducts.

CHAPTER 8

EXCRETORY SYSTEM

THE typical excretory system of adult digenetic Trematodes is
described as follows: There is a median excretory vesicle giving
off 2–6 main collecting tubes; these ramify into smaller tubes and
fine tubules, the blind distal ends of which are equipped with
flame cells. The vesicle is formed by the confluence of two

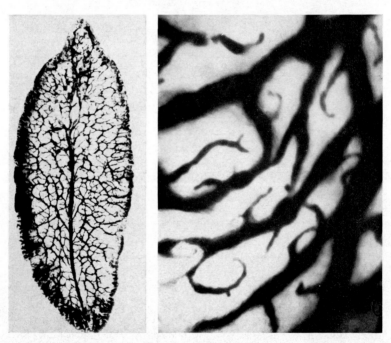

FIG. 34. Photograph of a liver fluke with the excretory system
injected with a dye, to show the degree of branching of the excretory
network. Right: Detail from the same preparation under high power
to show the terminal bifurcation of the tubules in the shape of a Y
(original).

78

initially distinct main tubes (as seen in the cercarial stage) and opens to the outside by a median pore at the posterior tip of the body.

In addition to this excretory network, another system of channels has been demonstrated in some digenetic Trematodes. Named by Looss "lymphatic system" at the beginning of the century, this system was mapped in detail by Willey (1930) for a number of species, but not for any of the Fasciolidae. Dawes (1946) outlining the structure of this in some Trematodes, added

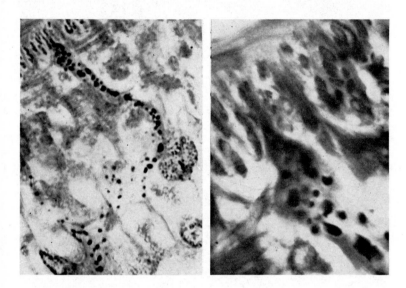

FIG. 35. End of an excretory tubule in a transverse section of an adult liver fluke fixed in Flemming's solution. The fat droplets are stained black. It can be seen how the end of the tubule or rather of the terminal cell appears to insert between the muscle fibres under the surface of the worm (original).

that it is absent "in other Digenerea" and stated that in the latter the fluid fills intercellular spaces which perhaps represent the rudiments of such a system.

The excretory system of *Fasciola hepatica* deviates from the typical pattern in several respects: the vesicle is very long (2/3 of body length) and only two short collecting tubes arise from it at its anterior end. Developmentally, however, it is the tubes that give rise to the bladder by fusion along 2/3 of their length (Kawana, 1940) (Fig. 36). Many, but not all of the smaller tubes open into the main collecting tubes; the majority open directly

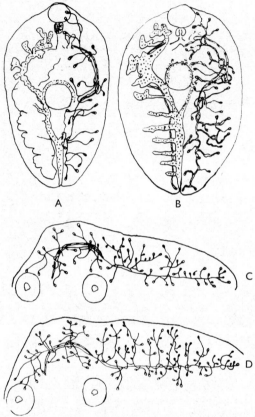

FIG. 36. Diagrams to show the gradual increase in complexity of the excretory network during the development of a metacercarium. A. 5th day after infection, the experimental host being the mouse. B. 10th day after infection. C. 11th day. D. 12th day (Kawana, 1940).

into the vesicle. Distally, the tubes anastomose and branch very profusely, more so near the dorsal body surface (Fig. 34).

The arrangement of the terminal excretory tubules, which open into the smaller branches of the collecting tubes can easily be made obvious. It is sufficient to inject some methylene blue solution with a micropipette, through the vesicle of a live liver fluke.

Under low magnification, it can then be seen that the excretory tubules, very numerous and situated predominantly near the dorsal surface, bifurcate always in the form of a Y. The branches end blindly with a slight distention at the end, where presumably the flame cells should be located (Fig. 34). It can also be seen that the anastomosing collecting tubules are of irregular width, expanding into small lacunae at intervals.

In histological section, the excretory and collecting tubules can be followed best after fixation in Flemming's solution. Numerous fat droplets in the tubes are thus stained black and so mark the course of the system. Often the terminal cell of a tubule sends cytoplasmic extensions towards the nearby cuticular epithelium. Figure 35 shows such a case. The extension proceeds into the muscular layers but does not actually come into contact with the basal membrane of the epithelium.

The facts that (a) the excretory tubules are concentrated near the body surface and (b) through their cytoplasmic extensions, they reach close to the surface, are probably of functional importance. There is evidence, in fact, that excess of iron taken up through the gut eventually reaches the cuticle. This appeared to be happening through the excretory tubules and/or the cells known as "myoblasts" (Pantelouris and Gresson, 1961; Pantelouris and Hale, 1962). In the case of the myoblasts, again a close connexion with the cuticle was recently demonstrated as already mentioned.

The excretory as well as the collecting network of tubes are all lined with cells, and are in no way simply confluent intercellular spaces. They do not therefore correspond to the lymphatic system described in some other Trematodes. In fact not only fat droplets but also vitamin C and iron are found within these cells which therefore may be actively involved in the transfer of materials into the lumen. It is noteworthy that this finding applies to the so-called collecting tubules as well as to the finer excretory tubules. In electron micrographs (Fig. 37) thin strips appear peeled off from the cell walls at one end but still anchored to it at the other; they give the impression of fingers or processes protruding into the lumen of the tubules. It is probable that the rather

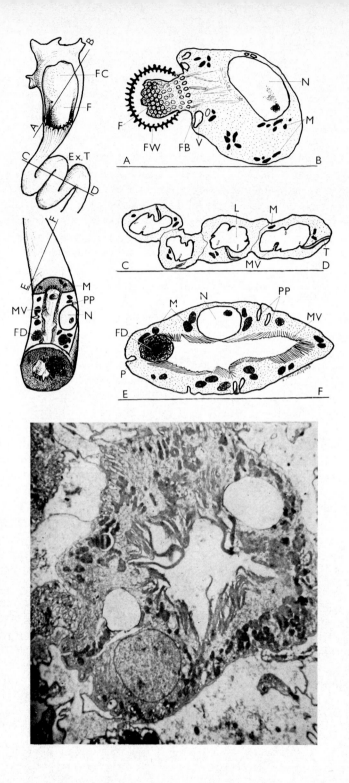

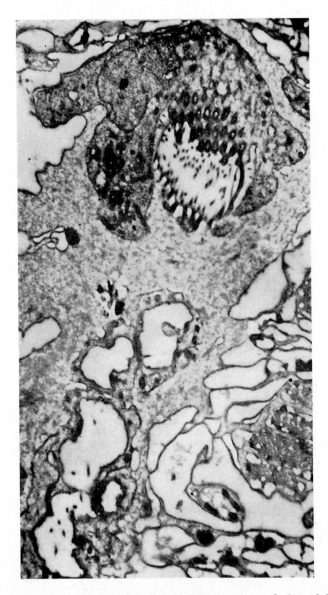

Fig. 37. The structure of the excretory system of the adult. (Diagrams by courtesy of L. T. Threadgold.) Top left: Diagrams to show the structure of an excretory tubule, and the appearance of sections along lines AB, CD and EF. Bottom left and above: Electron microphotographs of corresponding sections.

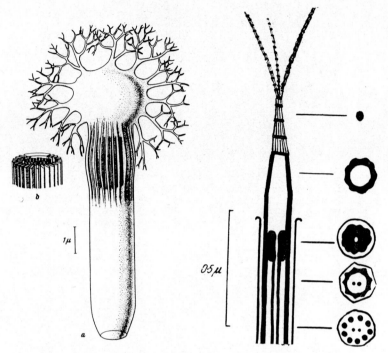

FIG. 38.   Left: Structure of the terminal excretory cell or solenocyte
of the miracidium. Right: structure of a single cilium of the flame-cell
and appearance of its transverse sections at different levels.
(Kümmel, 1959.)

large fat drops in the cells are released into the lumen by the cell
wall bursting locally, as remarked also by Prenant (1922), and that
the strips seen are ribbons of the erupted cell wall.

Workers generally have so far failed to observe flame-cells in
the tubules of the adult liver fluke, although these are easily seen
in the larval stages, and have been examined electron micro-
scopically by Kümmel (1959 and 1960) in sections of miracidia
(Fig. 38). The failure led Bugge (1929), Querner (1929) and
Stephenson (1947) to think that the flame tubules of the
cercarium are not represented in the adult. The existence of
flame-cells in the adult was simply assumed by others by analogy
with other Trematodes; also direct observation of flame cells by

Fraipont (1880) has been repeatedly cited. However, reference to Fraipont's paper shows that he did not examine specimens of *Fasciola hepatica* but was working on other Trematodes. Clegg (1947) did claim to have observed flame-cells; but his illustration is not clear and his observation, recorded in a thesis, is not widely known. More recently, however, unequivocal evidence of flame-cells was obtained by electron microscopy (Pantelouris and Threadgold, 1963) (Fig. 37). They are constructed on the same pattern as those described by Kümmel for the miracidium: the "flame" consists of numerous individual cilia all embedded in some ground material for most of their length and free only at the end; the transverse section of each cilium may show a lumen with a central filament or may be solid depending on the level of the section; finally, the sleeve in which the flame is enclosed shows a corrugated structure (Fig. 38). The flame cell can be described therefore as a "tubular cell" or solenocyte.

CHAPTER 9

CELL TYPES IN THE PARENCHYMA.
NERVOUS SYSTEM

THE parenchyma is made up in the main of large cells closely apposed to each other, so that their outline in section appears polygonal. In histological sections they appear to contain large vacuoles, but these are probably spaces left by the dissolution of the glycogen in the fixatives. In fact, in the whole cytoplasmic area of these cells and amidst the glycogen spaces, Björkman and Thorsell (1962) found numerous mitochondria, evidence of active metabolism (Fig. 39). The large glycogen reserves in these cells have been located by Örtner-Schonbach (1913) and Prenant (1922) as well as by many later workers. Threadgold noted that between adjacent cells of the parenchyma there is an electron-dense layer, much thicker than the interstitial material in other groups (Fig. 31).

Dispersed among the parenchymatic cells are a few other large cells with fine cytoplasmic extensions emerging from them (Fig. 40). Their exact nature is not known, but Alvarado (1951) considered them as ganglionic.

Cells of still another type give cytoplasmic extensions that are thick, tubular and bifurcate at some distance from the cell body (Fig. 40). Alvarado (1951) described how these extensions resemble a system of pipes meandering in between other cells, and was impressed by the variety of their staining reactions.

The parenchymatic cells, the basal membrane, myoblasts, dorso-ventral muscles, etc., are all surrounded by a network of fine fibres. Prenant (1922) and Alvarado (1951) have characterised the material of these fibres as "reticulin", but it is uncertain whether it is cellular or a secretion (Fig. 41).

Nervous System

The nervous system of the liver fluke has been described by Lang (1880), Bettendorf (1897) and Havet (1900) (Fig. 42).

Nerve cells can be demonstrated peripherally between the muscle fibres; they are found singly or in small groups, are oval and small, and give off 2–4 fibres. These proceed towards the epithelium and form a highly developed plexus.

Centrally there is one pair of ganglia on the sides of the pharynx and 6 nerves arising from each ganglion. Three of the six main nerves on each side proceed anteriorly; one is short and travels to

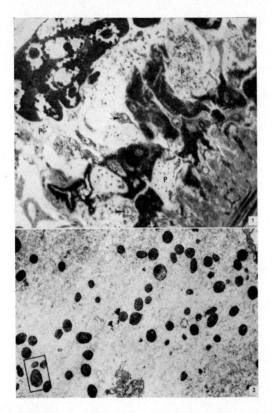

Fig. 39.   1. Section of liver fluke showing parenchymal cells (P) between the muscle layers (bottom right) and a yolk gland (upper left). The granules in the parenchyma cells are mitochondria, and the arrows point to nuclei.

2. Part of a parenchymal cell under the electron microscope, showing the mitochondria of different sizes (Björkman and Thorsell, 1962) (see also Figs. 40 and 41).

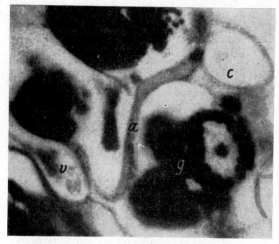

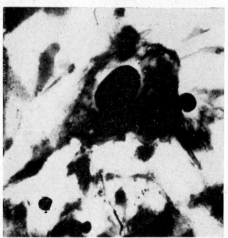

Fig. 40. Top: Detail from the parenchyma, stained by the silver carbonate technique. *g*, yolk cell. *v*, vacuolated cell with its peri-cellular reticulin net. *c*, "cell with large extensions", *a*, being one of these extensions (Alvarado, 1951).

Bottom: One of the "large cells" described by Alvarado, again stained by the silver carbonate method.

the corresponding edge of the body, whilst the other two are directed posteriorly. Of the latter two, the thicker one comes to lie near the ventral surface and extends parallel to the main axis of the body towards the posterior end of the body.

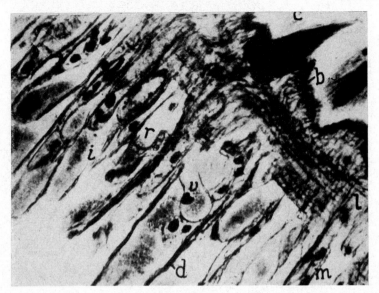

Fig. 41.   Part of transverse section stained with silver carbonate to demonstrate the reticulin fibres.
c, cuticular epithelium. *b*, basal membrane. *r*, peri-cellular network of reticulin. *i*, cell inclusions. *v*, vesiculated cell. *d*, dorso-ventral muscle. *m*, myoblast. *l*, longitudinal muscles delimited their reticulin sheath (Alvarado, 1951).

Numerous small lateral nerves arise from these six main longitudinal nerves.

Bettendorf described only 4 pairs of main nerves. He also demonstrated two plexuses in the suckers and considered the superficial plexus as sensory and the deeper, connected with the ventral nerves, as motor. He further described piriform sense cells which receive a nerve fibre at the one end, and at the other form sensory papillae on the body surface. He specifically mentioned these structures in the liver fluke, although his best preparations were from other Trematodes.

G

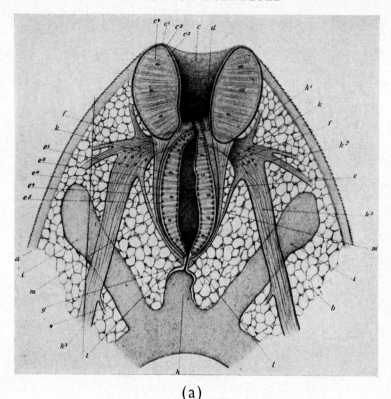

(a)

FIG. 42. The nervous system of the liver fluke.

Left. A diagram by Sommer (1880) of the anterior part of the worm at a horizontal section through the mouth and pharynx showing the central part of the nervous system. Right, photograph of a similar stained section, at a more dorsal level, showing clearly the commissure around the dorsal half of the pharynx.

c, oral sucker, showing in section the cuticle c_1 and the three layers of fibres c_2, c_3 and c_4. f, protractor muscle of pharynx.

d, valve between sucker and pharynx e. Layers of muscle fibres in the pharynx include: e_2, inner circular; e_3, radial with some ganglionic cells amongst them; e_4, outer circular, and e_5, longitudinal.

b, the gut, connecting to the pharynx by a very narrow part, g. k, k, the two "pharyngeal" ganglia, connected by a pharyngeal commissure, $comm$. k_1, k_2, k_3 anterior, posterior outer and posterior inner nerves. A branch of the latter to the cirrus pouch is shown, marked by an asterisk*.

m, side commissures connecting the pharyngeal ganglion of each side to another smaller "lower pharyngeal ganglion", l.

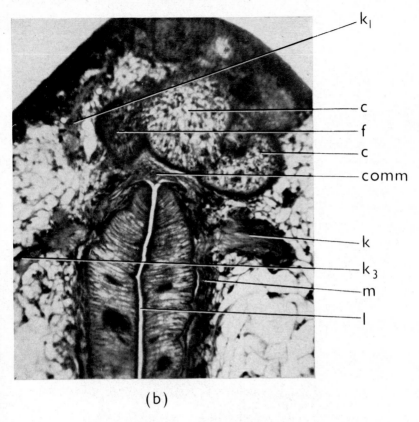

(b)

Acetylcholinesterase has been detected in liver fluke material by Bacq and Oury (1937), Chance and Mansour (1953), and Sekardi and Ehrlich (1962). Atebrin, a substance that has found some use as an anthelminthic, and caffeine inhibit the enzyme. Acetylcholine in the presence of either of these inhibitors or of eserine kills liver flukes *in vitro*.

The "deganglionated preparation" of a liver fluke obtained by cutting off the cephalic cone of the worm maintains its rhythmic contractions for about 2 hr. Various sympathicomimetic amines (including adrenaline), eserine, acetylcholine and carbaminoylcholine chloride, all have an inhibitory effect on the preparation (Chance and Mansour, 1953).

CHAPTER 10

REPRODUCTIVE SYSTEM

THE testes are two convoluted tubes spread in the parenchyma over a central oval area roughly corresponding to one-third of the whole body. They are located one behind the other, and a fine sperm duct from each leads forward to a joint seminal vesicle; from this a short ejaculatory duct traverses the muscular, retractable copulatory organ or cirrus. The cirrus can be retracted into a cirrus sac or pouch (Fig. 43).

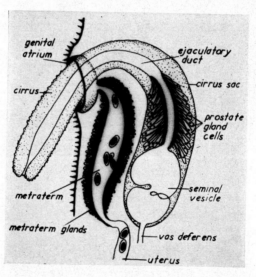

FIG. 43. Diagram to show the relationships of the terminal reproductive organs of Digenerean Trematodes (Noble, E. R. and Noble, G. A., *Parasitology*. Kimpton, London, 1961) (see also Fig. 25C).

The single ovary is branched and situated on the left of the midline behind the ventral sucker. The short oviduct joins the anterior vitelline duct. At the junction the anterior vitelline

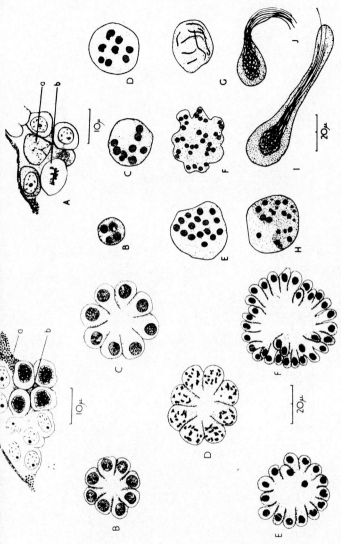

Fig. 44. Left: The normal stages of spermatogenesis. *A*, lining of tubule. *a*, globule. *b*, tetrad of tertiary spermatogonia. *B*, 8-cell primary spermatocyte morula. *C*, the same after growth. *D*, reduction division at metaphase, 8 cells. *E*, 16-cell morula of secondary spermatocytes. *F*, 32-cell morula of early spermatids.

Right: Abnormal forms appearing after maintenance of the worm in unsuitable media. *A*, lining of a tubule. *a*, abnormal spermatogonia. *b*, metaphase in a primary spermatogonium. *B*, abnormal tertiary spermatogonia, group of four nuclei. *C–J*, abnormal morulae and spermatids (Clegg, 1947).

duct distends into an ootype; this is followed by the uterus, also convoluted, which opens to the outside by a small pore next to the cirrus opening. Both the male and female pores open into a small and shallow atrium, reaching the surface by a gonopore.

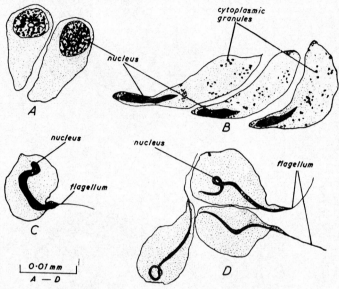

FIG. 45. Spermateleosis, the final stages of spermatogenesis in the liver fluke. *A*, young spermatids. The pointed ends of the cells are directed towards the blastophore. *B*, spermatids. The distal ends of the cells and their nuclei have undergone a process of elongation. *C*, spermatid. A flagellum is now visible at the distal end of the cell. *D*, late spermatids. The nucleus of each cell has become thread-like and the flagellum is growing out from the distal end of the cell (Gresson, 1957).

At the junction of vitelline duct and oviduct there is the beginning of still another fine duct, known as Laurer's canal, which opens separately by a minute pore on the dorsal body surface. In addition there is a whole cluster of gland cells, forming the Mehli's gland, surrounding the ootype (Fig. 48). There is a one-way uterine valve between ootype and uterus. Some structural and functional details of this female genital complex are in dispute.

The segment between the anterior vitelline duct and valve is considered a single structure by some authors and is called by

Stephenson (1947c), central chamber of Mehli's gland and by Rao (1959), ootype or central chamber. Yosufzai (1953a), on the other hand, distinguished a proximal elliptical chamber and pictured the oviduct opening into it, and a proximal uterus.

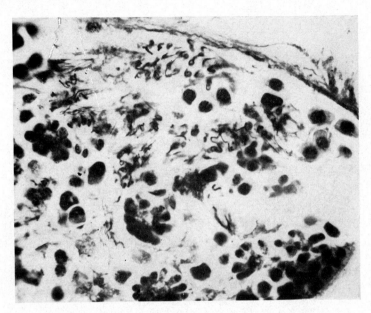

FIG. 46.   Transverse section through a testis tubule, showing various stages of spermatogenesis. Compare with Fig. 44 (original).

Mehli's gland has no duct but its secretion presumably infiltrates through the cells of the walls of both the elliptical chamber and/or the proximal uterus.

Abnormalities occasionally observed include lobulate and bilateral ovary, and even absence of vitellaria and testes (Healy, 1955b; Gállego-Berenguer, 1952).

Spermatogenesis

Essentially, spermatogenesis in the liver fluke does not diverge from the normal metazoan pattern (Figs. 44 to 46).

In a transverse section of the testis, the primary spermatogonia are at the periphery in clusters 2–3 cells deep. Each spermatogonium grows and divides to two secondary spermatogonia.

Clegg (1957) states that each primary spermatogonium divides into two cells of which only one is a secondary spermatogonium, whilst the other is a primordial cell that will in time develop to give another primordial cell and a primary spermatogonium. Each

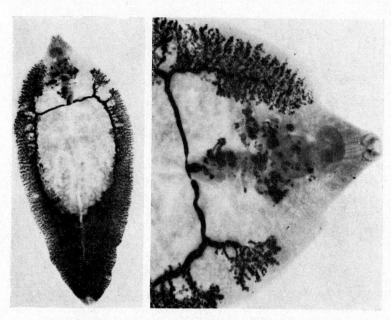

FIG. 47. The system of vitelline glands and ducts, and the female genital ducts, made visible in a whole mount of an adult liver fluke by staining by Smyth's catechol method (original). Compare with Fig. 25A.

secondary spermatogonium gives rise to a tetrad of tertiary spermatogonia. After another division the resulting eight primary spermatocytes form a "morula"; according to Yosufzai (1952), the eight cells of the morula are all attached to a central disk which may itself contain a nucleus-like body.

A meiotic division follows and sixteen secondary spermatocytes are formed; these still remain attached to the central blastophore and give rise in turn by a further division to a bundle of 32 spermatids. To become a mature spermatozoon the spermatid elongates as a whole but the nucleus elongates even more than the

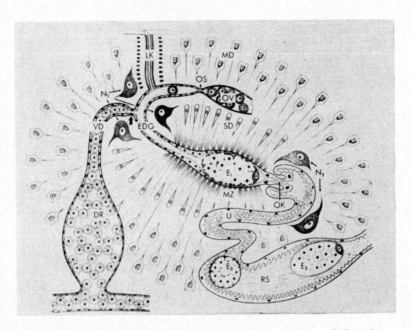

Fɪɢ. 48. The female genital complex, or oogenotype, of *Fasciola hepatica* according to Gönnert (1962), to whom we owe a most thorough re-examination of the problem. *DR*, vitelline reservoir. E_1, egg in the ootype with the beginnings of shell formation. E_2, egg in the upper uterus, confluence of shell droplets completed. E_3, egg in the uterus, shell formation completed. *EDG*, ovovitelloduct. *LK*, Laurer's canal. *MD*, mucous cells of Mehli's gland. *MZ*, openings of the cells of Mehli's gland. N_1, nerve plexus at the confluence of the vitelline duct, *VD*, and the ovovitelloduct. The arrow indicates the presence of a sphincter at the end of the vitelline duct. N_2, nerve plexus around the beginning of the uterus. Nerve plexus 1 comprises four to five cells, nerve plexus 2 consists of only two cells. *O*, ootype with a valve at the end, *OK*. *OV*, oviduct with a sphincter, *OS*. *RS*, receptaculum seminis. *SD*, cells of Mehli's gland producing a serous secretion (Stephenson's inner eosinophilic zone of the gland). *U*, uterus.

rest. In fact, the nucleus becomes thread-like and eventually coiled, and its distal end protrudes out of the cytoplasm though still retaining a fine cytoplasmic sheath. The main part of the cytoplasm differentiates to a flagellum. Nucleus and flagellum now become disentangled from the residual cytoplasm of the spermatid. There is no middle or neck or centrosome according to Gresson (1957), despite claims to the opposite by Yosufzai. Whilst it is usually stated that the 32 spermatozoa remain in a bundle together for some time, Hendelberg (1962) showed that the bundles contain spermatids and not spermatozoa. He also convincingly demonstrated that the spermatozoa are biflagellate, the two flagella connected in parallel so as to appear like a compound flagellum. Biflagellate spermatozoa are the rule amongst Digenea.

All spermatogenetic stages may be found together in any single lobe of the testis, intermingled with groups of small globules or masses of cytoplasm without nucleus. The spermatozoa are intensely Feulgen-positive (Bogomoleva, 1956) but also carry some ribonucleic acid.

The Yolk Glands

Each of the two small vitelline ducts entering the pear-shaped vitelline reservoir on the midline leads distally to one longitudinal yolk-collecting duct on each side of the body, running practically parallel to the body outline. Into these two main longitudinal ducts open innumerable short branching tubules from the yolk follicles, the distribution of which can be seen in Fig. 26.

The vitelline cells originate from the cells of the follicle walls, from which they become detached as they mature. When still immature, they have a clear cytoplasm, and occasionally cell divisions may be seen. Stephenson has seen about six chromosomes per cell in such cases and therefore considers them as haploid cells. Two types of cytoplasmic inclusion subsequently form in large quantities; yolk globules and smaller basophilic granules described by some as "shell granules". These, according to Smyth and Clegg (1959) and Romanini (1947), contain protein and phenol and the enzymes necessary to effect the eventual transformation of these substances to a tanned protein.

Romanini (1947) Ranzoli (1955 and 1956) and Rao (1959a and b; 1960) found that the vitelline cells give a PAS-positive reaction removable by amylase, hence indicating the presence of glycogen; but this reaction is absent from the still immature cells near the periphery of the vitelline glands. Azure Schiff-positive granules are also described.

When the vitelline cells enter the vitelline reservoir they begin to discharge both types of globules. In Yosufzai's description, these globules and unbroken vitelline cells proceed to the elliptical chamber. The ova arrive via the oviduct, and the hyaline secretion of the Mehli's gland also collects here (Fig. 48).

Mehli's Gland or Shell-gland

This consists peripherally of numerous pear-shaped basophilic unicellular glands; thin cytoplasmic funnels from these converge to the centre, and traverse the cells of the ootype wall to open into the ootype independently (Gönnert, 1962).

By silver staining techniques, Yosufzai claimed to have detected a hyaline secretion between these cytoplasmic funnels. Rao (1959, 1960) found that the secretion is Azur Schiff-negative but PAS-positive; while because of the eosinophilic staining of the cytoplasmic funnels Stephenson concluded that the secretion must be alkaline.

Smyth (1951) also found that this gland gives no positive reaction for proteins, phenols and phenolases, in contrast to the egg-shell granules of the yolk cells. (This point is important in connexion with theories of the origin of the egg shell.) He is also cited (Johri, 1957) as having confirmed the presence of PAS-positive but non-glycogen material (mucoprotein, mucopolysaccharide or glycoprotein).

Formation of Egg Yolk and Egg Shell

In the elliptical chamber the released yolk globules and also the shell granules cluster around the egg. The secretion from Mehli's gland forms a hyaline shell around the egg; after this the egg proceeds through the proximal uterus and the valve into the distal uterus. It is here that it meets spermatozoa for the first time so that fertilization must be taking place through the shell. In this conclusion Yosufzai concurred with certain earlier authors: Blumberg (1911), Sommer (1880) Looss (1885) and Schubman (1905).

However, most authors disagree with this description. Stephenson described the release of yolk globules and of the polyphenol granules from the vitelline cells as occurring in the uterus beyond the valve and in the presence of spermatozoa. In fact he commented on the penetration of spermatozoa into eggs and/or vitelline cells indiscriminately. Kouri *et al.* (1931) attributed the formation of the egg shell to the vitelline granules.

A third group of workers (Henneguy, 1902 and 1906; Tyzzer, 1918; Dawes, 1940) believed that both Mehli's secretion and the granules from the vitelline cells take part in the formation of the egg shell.

Smyth (1954) and Smyth and Clegg (1959) have settled this point (Fig. 49). The protein and diphenol found in the "egg-shell

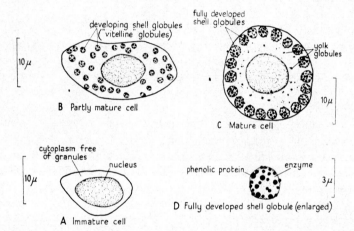

Fig. 49. The stages of vitellogenesis in the yolk cells of the liver fluke (Smyth, 1954).

granules" together with suitable oxidase constitute a system that leads in the presence of oxygen, to the formation of a quinone from the diphenol and then to the complexing of the protein with the quinone, i.e. the tanning of the proteins to form the sclerotin cover of the eggs. This change is effected as the egg passes along the uterus and Stephenson suggested that oxidization is due to a tissue haemoglobin. However, in freshly obtained flukes a few most recent eggs will be found still unstained. Some tanning occurs if the worm is kept *in vitro* in aerobic conditions; but this is prevented by horse serum (Clegg, 1957). Smyth demonstrated the presence of this system in the granules by incubating frozen-dried sections with 0·2 per cent catechol at 40°C; within 2 min the granules in the vitelline cells become yellow, later pink and, if left for some hours, brown.

Mansour (1957b and 1958) made a study of the phenol-oxidase from the liver fluke and found it different in several respects from that of some other invertebrates.

The fact that Mehli's gland is negative for protein, phenols and phenolase, whilst the egg-shell granules are positive, means that these granules contribute to the egg shell; but it does not exclude the possibility that Mehli's secretion may also contribute a membrane around the egg possibly impregnated later by the other materials.

Oogenesis

The oogonia have a large nucleus with little cytoplasm at the periphery. The fine channels of endoplasmic reticulum seen in the cytoplasm connect with both the nuclear envelope and the plasma membrane in these cells (Gresson, 1962). Yosufzai (1952) claimed that the nucleus extrudes material into the cytoplasm, to such an extent that the former loses all its chromatin. He also described extrusion of the contents of the one or two nucleoli, occurring whilst the oogonium grows to become a primary oocyte. Golgi elements (in the form of granules and rods at one pole of the nucleus in the young oocyte, and in the form of granules dispersed throughout the cytoplasm in the mature oocyte) were also described by the same author.

Henneguy (1906) and Sanderson (1953) failed to see a polar body or a second maturation division. The latter author further believed that the sperm entering the egg remains outside the spindle area (already formed in some cases), and that no male pronucleus is formed; the diploid number of female chromosomes seemed to form two distinct nuclei which subsequently fused. On this evidence, the process would be one of pseudogamous gynogenesis. However, in a later study (1959) the same author reported that she was able now to see the expulsion of two polar nuclei, so that the gynogenetic theory had to be abandoned.

The Feulgen-positive material is distributed uniformly as fine filaments throughout the germinal vesicle of the oocyte; this enabled Govaert (1953a and b, 1954, 1955 and 1960) to study the DNA content quantitatively by Feulgen staining. His conclusion is that the DNA content of the oocyte remains constant throughout oogenesis. The oocyte nucleus does not give the Millon reaction for protein, in contrast to the nuclei of yolk cells before the formation of yolk granules (Fautrez, 1958).

Fertilization

Although it has been suggested that copulation may take place through the Laurer's canal, it seems more probable that, normally, the cirrus is inserted into the uterus or at least into the genital atrium. Again, it is not clear whether this process is used for self-fertilization or whether cross-fertilization is the rule. That self-fertilization occurs has been shown beyond doubt. Hughes (1959), for example, obtained fertile eggs from a solitary fluke in an experimentally infected rabbit.

The sperm ascends from the uterus to the ootype (Gönnert, 1962). Several spermatozoa may enter one egg (leaving their tails behind); of these sperms one fuses with the oocyte or ovum whilst the others reach the vitelline cells of the egg where they degenerate.

By the time of fertilization the ovum has gone through the first maturation division; the second maturation division takes place after fertilization (Yosufzai, 1953).

Marzullo *et al.* (1957) failed to demonstrate histochemically the presence of glycogen and phosphatases in the egg. They explain this by the formation of complex substances and by the small quantities involved respectively.

Chromosome Numbers

The diploid chromosome number of the liver fluke is given as 12 by some authors (Schellenberg, 1911; John, 1953) and as 20 by others (Clegg, 1957; Sanderson, 1953). On the other hand, Henneguy (1907) was able to count 6–8 chromosomes in the oocyte, while Schubman (1905) counted 8–16 and 9–14.

CHAPTER 11

METABOLIC STUDIES

OUR knowledge of the metabolism of *Fasciola hepatica* is fragmentary. Whatever is known is based on histological, cytochemical and chemical tests and analyses on parasites removed from their habitat and on a few experiments *in vitro*.

Carbohydrate Metabolism

Carbohydrate Stores

Glycogen is the main source of energy for all helminths living in an oxygen-poor environment (von Brand, 1926). The amount of glycogen in the liver fluke is given, on the basis of chemical determinations, as 3·1 per cent of fresh and 15 per cent of dry weight by Flury and Leeb (1926), and as 3·7 per cent and 21 per cent by Weinland and Brand (1926). For comparison, *Fasciola gigantica* was found to have 5·4 per cent and 25·3 per cent of glycogen falling to 3·5 per cent and 15·3 per cent after starvation (Goil, 1961).

The glycogen is localized in the parenchyma, the mature yolk cells and (to a lesser extent) in the testes (Örtner-Schonbach, 1913; Semichon, 1933; Dawes and Müller, 1957). It is also found in the mature oocytes but disappears after fertilization; this may indicate that it is used up to release the energy required in the maturation divisions. Glycogen contained in the yolk cells becomes enclosed within the egg, to supply the needs of the various larval stages. Ginetskiskaya (1960) detected it histochemically in the parenchyma of cercaria of various Trematodes. The highest concentration is in the suckers and the walls of the excretory vesicle, and in the case of furcocercaria, in the "caudal bodies". Although the cercaria studied did not include those of *Fasciola,* it would be reasonable to assume the same for this species. The same author believes that this glycogen is not used up to provide energy for the cercarium's free movement but only or mainly for the penetration into the host. She made no suggestion as to the source of energy utilized for cercarial movement.

Starvation reduces the amount of glycogen in the parenchyma and muscle layers of the adult, but the glycogen of the uterus appears to be spared (von Brand and Mercado, 1961).

In addition to glycogen, helminths generally carry varying amounts of glucose, a reducing sugar, and of trehalose, a non-reducing sugar; however *Fasciola* seems to contain only traces of the latter (Fairburn, 1958).

Experiments in Absence of Oxygen

The end products of the anaerobic metabolism of carbohydrates are fatty acids, and the abundance of fat droplets in the fluke's excretory tubes is evidence that this parasite is anaerobic; certain experiments however suggest that oxygen, if available, is utilized to some extent. The direct information available concerning the use of carbohydrates by the liver fluke is due to the investigations of Weinland and Brand (1926), van Grembergen (1949) and Mansour (1959). (The latter worked with flukes collected in the Gulf area of U.S.A., and suspected that they may be hybrids of *F. hepatica* and *gigantica*).

Weinland and von Brand obtained a reduction by 15–37 per cent of the glycogen content of halved flukes by maintaining them for 6 hours in an atmosphere free of CO_2; anything from 0·29 to 0·59 mg of CO_2 were produced per specimen. Increased oxygenation did not affect this quantity.

In some of his experiments, Mansour kept specimens in Hédon-Fleig saline without glucose in an atmosphere of nitrogen. The total carbohydrate content fell from 220–180 to 97–84 μ moles/g of wet weight in six hours. Overnight starvation reduced the initial carbohydrate to about half and also reduced the amounts utilized in the six hours to only 18–35 μ moles.

In the presence of glucose but still anaerobically, 110–195 μ moles/g w.wt. of the sugar were utilized; this not only covered immediate metabolic requirements but brought about an increase of total polysaccharide stores by 20–44 μ moles. In this respect there was no significant difference between starved and non-starved worms.

Experiments in the Presence of Oxygen

In Mansour's experiments 35–42 m moles of oxygen /g w. wt. were utilized in 3 hr in the absence of glucose. Addition of glucose to the medium does not appreciably change oxygen uptake, or affect the respiratory quotient which stays at $1 \cdot 65$–$2 \cdot 2$. The CO_2 released amounted to 50–76 m moles. This high ratio of CO_2 to O_2 indicates that about half the CO_2 released is produced anaerobically. Nor does the presence of oxygen decrease the amount of glucose utilized.

The conclusion of Grembergen (1949), that glucose does not stimulate aerobic metabolism and oxygen utilization was thus confirmed. Grembergen had also found that even increased partial pressure of oxygen fails to increase oxygen uptake. His experiments were carried out on homogenized fluke tissue suspended in saline.

In contrast, using intact flukes, Harnisch (1932a and b) could detect some slight increase of uptake with raised oxygen pressure.

Grembergen's estimate of oxygen uptake was 400–540 ml/hr/g wt. while Harnisch's was only 13–28 ml/15 hr/g. Expressed in ml O_2 per gram wet weight per hour, these measurements become:

Intact flukes in Hédon-Fleig (Mansour)	269–314
Homogenate in saline (Grembergen)	400–540
Intact flukes in saline (Harnisch)	92–112.

Further evidence for the ability of the fluke to utilize oxygen was obtained by Rohrbacher (1957). In a pyruvate solution *in vitro* the parasite survived for 6 days, compared to 2 days under strict anaerobic conditions. Glutamic acid also extends survival to 4 days.

Enzymes involved in aerobic metabolism, small as this may be, are present and similar to those present in mammalian tissues, judging by the results of tests carried out by Grembergen (1949): succinic acid raises or stabilizes oxygen utilization; malic acid and malonic acid act antagonistically; therefore, succinic dehydrogenase is present. Similarly oxygen utilization is enhanced by methylene blue, α-glycerophosphoric acid, glutamic acid, dinitrophenol and *p*-phenylene diamine; this indicates the presence of cytochrome oxidase.

H

New light was shed on this question by more recent investigations. Von Brand and Mercado (1961) demonstrated that starved flukes kept in a medium containing glucose and 30 per cent serum resynthesize their lost carbohydrate. Bryant and Williams (1962) kept adult liver flukes in Hédon-Fleig solution to which they added carbon-labelled glucose or succinic acid. When they fixed the tissues in alcohol, homogenized and collected the supernatant, this contained about 10 per cent of the radioactivity in the case of glucose, but much less in the case of succinate. By chromatographic separation and autoradiography these workers demonstrated in the first case the presence of radioactive intermediates of glycolysis; in the second case they demonstrated intermediates of the Krebs cycle (Figs. 50, 52 and Table 6). Fluke homogenate metabolizes labelled succinate, but not labelled glucose (Bryant and Smith, 1963).

TABLE 6. PER CENT INCORPORATION OF RADIOACTIVITY BY LIVER FLUKES FROM CARBON-LABELLED GLUCOSE AND SUCCINIC ACID IN THE MEDIUM INTO SOLUBLE INTERMEDIATES EXCLUDING RESIDUAL SUBSTRATE (BRYANT AND WILLIAMS, 1962)

	Glucose		Succinic acid	
	Adult	Miracidia	Adult	Miracidia
Associated with glycolytic activity:				
Hexose phosphate and				
Phosphoenol pyruvate	15	21		
Alanine	10	26		
Lactate	18	30	30	0
Associated with Krebs cycle activity:				
Succinate	17	0		
Fumarate	1	0	3	
Malate	4	0	24	100*
Citrate	4	0	11	
Glutamate	10	0	7	
Gamma-aminobutyrate	6	0	10	
Disaccharide	3	7		

* This represents only 1 per cent of the original radioactivity, the remainder was recovered as unchanged substrate.

It is concluded that both the glycolytic series of reactions from glucose to pyruvic acid, and the tricarboxylic acid cycle (Krebs cycle) are in evidence in the adult.

The position regarding the Krebs cycle is different in the miracidia however. If succinate is supplied in excess, they

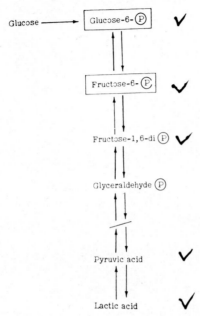

FIG. 50. A diagram showing in an abbreviated form the chain of glycolytic reactions, with the intermediate metabolites detected in the adult liver fluke by Bryant and Williams (1962) ticked off.

utilize it to malate, i.e. they carry the enzymes, succinic dehydrogenase and fumarase. But this accumulates, i.e. the miracidia do not form from it the oxalacetic acid which enters in the beginning of the Krebs cycle. Such a gradual building up of the full enzymatic complement from stage to stage appears to be widespread in helminths (Vernberg and Hunter, 1960) (See Fig. 51).

As mentioned earlier on, non-volatile fatty acids and liquids, as well as traces of volatile fatty acids, are the end-products of carbohydrate metabolism in *Fasciola hepatica*; in the case, however, of the specimens used by Mansour (1958, 1959) the volatile acids

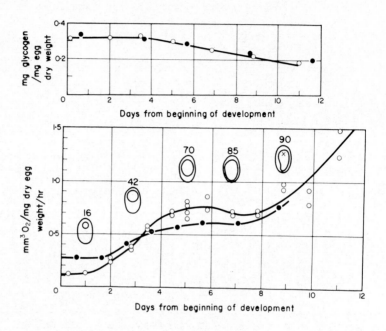

Fig. 51. The gradual increase in metabolic rate in the developing egg (Horstmann, 1962).

A. Glycogen content of eggs of *Fasciola hepatica* during the development of the miracidium at 25°C. Circles, eggs collected from the gall bladder of the host. Dots, eggs removed from mature flukes.

B. Oxygen utilization of eggs during early development at 25°C. Numbers by the eggs indicate the length of the enclosed embryo in μ. Oxygen is essential for the development of the eggs, which can be stopped by blowing nitrogen through the culture vessel for one hour. It was also found that oxygen utilization is higher in the light than in darkness.

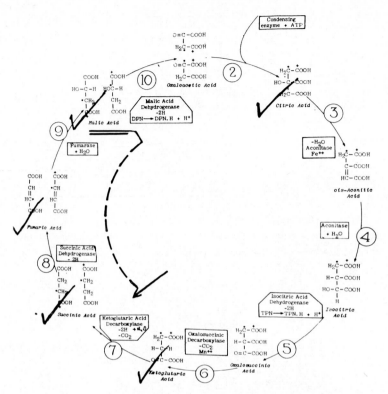

Fig. 52. Diagram showing the Krebs cycle with the enzymes shown to exist in the adult liver fluke ticked off. The arc from the arrow to the two parallel lines marks the portion of the Krebs cycle that has been shown to exist in the miracidium (from the results of Bryant and Williams, 1962).

(propionic and acetic in the ratio of 3:1) by far exceeded lactic acid, the latter representing only 4 per cent of the products. It may be noted here that the level of acetone, acetoacetic acid, β-hydroxybutyric acid and ketone bodies is stated to be higher in cattle harbouring liver flukes than in healthy animals (Salutini, 1959).

Stimulation of muscular activity by serotonin increases the proportion of lactic acid by 2–6 times. By further analysing the effect of serotonin with cell-free homogenates, Mansour (1959) concluded that it stimulates both glycogenolysis and glycolysis, as epinephrine does in higher animals.

Other Metabolites

Fats are also utilized by the parasite to some extent. In the experiments of Weinland and Brand (1926), it was found that not only the stores of glycogen, but also the ether-extractable components of the parasite were reduced from 1·48–2·33 per cent of fresh weight to 1·24–1·86 per cent after 6 hr in saline in an atmosphere free of CO_2. A corresponding increase of fat content of the medium (estimated by addition of H_2SO_4 and extraction with ether) was also obtained.

Protein makes up 58 per cent of the dry weight of *Fasciola hepatica* (Weinland and Brand, 1926), and a large amount is also synthesized in the enormous number of oocytes and spermatozoa.

TABLE 7. TRANSAMINASE ACTIVITY OF LIVER FLUKE HOMOGENATES (DOUGHERTY, 1952)

Aminoacid	Mean	Aminoacid	Mean
Aspartic acid	207	Tyrosine	32
Isoleucine	201	Methionine	24
Leucine	179	Proline	14
Valine	141	Tryptophane	3
Arginine	104	Lysine	0
Alanine	95	Cystine	0
Phenylalanine	39		

(The figures are means expressed as μ moles of glutamic acid formed from a-ketoglutaric acid per gram of fresh tissue per hour)

Expressing protein content in terms of total nitrogen as per cent of dry weight, Goil (1958) reached an estimate of 10·64 per cent for *Fasciola gigantica* (and smaller figures for some other Trematodes). Both Dougherty (1952) and Maekawa and Kushibe (1956) detected several aminoacids in non-hydrolysed extracts of liver fluke (with particularly high values for glutamic acid, aspartic and valine); however, sulphur-containing aminoacids (methionine and cystine) are stated to be absent.

The large amounts of glutamic acid are correlated with the presence of transaminase activity, detected by Dougherty (1952) in homogenates of whole liver flukes in Krebs–Ringer phosphate solution (Table 7). In the transaminase reaction glutamic acid acts as the acceptor of the amino group.

Excretory Products

Von Brand and Weinland (1924) were the first to draw attention to the fat drops detectable with osmic acid fixatives in the lumen of the tubules. Incidentally they also found fat droplets at places on the testis sheath, but not in the yolk (as it had been claimed by Sommer, 1880). Stephenson (1947) ascertained by histochemical tests that the globules contain no cholesterol, cholesterides or lipids. Therefore, he concluded, the droplets contain no lipid material of the kind found in the bile. It is presumed that the droplets consist of products of anaerobic glycolysis.

Stephenson also discovered that the walls of the excretory tubules and a "submuscular cell layer" are rich in vitamin C which gives the silver nitrate reaction, but could suggest no explanation of this phenomenon. Recently, Pantelouris and Hale (1962) correlated the presence of the vitamin with that of iron. On mapping the distribution of the two substances they found that it overlaps. The iron was detected in these experiments by autoradiography (after ingestion by the oral sucker of Fe59) and by the Prussian blue test; the vitamin was located by its silver nitrate reaction. The overlapping is explained by the role of vitamin C in maintaining the iron in a soluble form to facilitate its excretion.

The main excretory products are carbon monoxide, hydrogen sulphide, ammonia and the short chain fatty acids (Flury and Leeb, 1926).

The main nitrogen-containing excretory products were identified by Goil (1958) by analysis of a non-nutrient culture medium in which the worms were kept aerobically (but under axenic conditions) for 12 hr at 37°C: ammonia excreted in 2 hr represented 1·41–2·51 per cent of the total nitrogen, but uric acid only 0·038–0·10 per cent. No urea or creatinine were found. Florkin and Duchateau (1943) failed to find enzymes that would break down the uric acid further; hence the uric acid forming from the degradation of purines is excreted as such.

Respiratory Pigment

In evaluating the results of *in vitro* studies, the possibility should be kept in mind that, in its natural location, the parasite may be able to make some use of the oxygen carried by the ingested oxyhaemoglobin. There is evidence of this happening in the case of hookworms (Wells, 1931). However, Weinland and Brand calculated that even if each fluke used up 0·001 per cent of the host liver per month, the oxygen obtained would only supply 1 per cent of the oxygen required by mammalian tissues.

Rohrbacher considered that there is sufficient oxygen in the bile ducts (at least as long as these are not yet calcified) — though not in the gall bladder. Diffusion through the worm's body surface should be fully adequate, he estimated, because of the large surface to volume ratio of the thin leaf-like worm; the surface of a fluke is about 300 mm² and the volume 100 mm³.

The parasite contains a red pigment which Stephenson (1947) and Grembergen (1949) classified as a myoglobin. Homogenates of the worm's tissue buffered in phosphate and seen through the spectroscope give an absorption band at 580–581 mμ, which is typical for oxyhaemoglobin, and one at 540–543 mμ, which is typical for "muscular haemoglobin" or myoglobin. Neither of these bands is due to haemoglobin in the gut contents. In fact, Grembergen found that the homogenate from flukes with empty gut gave clearer bands than homogenate from worms with full gut. In addition, similar bands are given by homogenates of tissue of another Trematode, *Dicrocoelium lanceolatum,* where the gut is non-ramifying and therefore samples definitely free of gut contents can be prepared; the same applies to *Telorchis robustus* (Wharton, 1941), a Trematode parasite in the gut of the turtle.

Working with *Fasciola gigantica* from buffaloes, Goil (1961) concluded that, in this species at least, the pigment is not a myoglobin but a haemoglobin; at the same time it appears to differ from the haemoglobin of the host.

Whatever the exact nature of the pigment, there seems to be no doubt about its occurrence in the tissues of the parasite; but there is no indication whatsoever about its possible importance in aerobic metabolism.

Iron and Copper Metabolism

Both the presence of a "myoglobin" in the tissues and the fact that the parasite must be ingesting large amounts of liver tissue and some blood (both materials rich in ferritin or haemoglobin) raise the question of iron metabolism. In particular, it may be asked whether iron is absorbed to any extent from the gut, and if so how is it eliminated to prevent its accumulation in the parasite. Furthermore, the extent to which the parasite causes iron loss and anaemia in the host, is also of obvious importance and merits investigation.

Stephenson (1947) was the first to investigate the fate of ingested haemoglobin. He first established that the brown pigment usually filling the gut is a haematin, and that it corresponds to about a six-fold concentration of blood. By following the changes in the ingested blood spectroscopically, he concluded that haemolysis starts a few hours after ingestion and results in the production of brown granules of acid haematin. To reach this stage, the oxyhaemoglobin ingested is reduced to haemoglobin before haemolysis. Grembergen (1950) added methaemoglobin to this sequence.

It does not follow from these observations that all the iron in the ingested food is eliminated as haematin with the faeces. In fact, Pantelouris and Gresson (1960) found that the fluke tissues can be labelled by the "injection" into the gut through the oral sucker of ferric iron-59 in solution, or of iron-labelled blood. Pantelouris and Hale (1962) further produced evidence that the excess iron is eliminated through both the excretory system and the cuticle and also that its localization in the tissues overlaps that of vitamin C (Figs. 53–54). This overlap may facilitate the disposal of iron, as vitamin C forms soluble compounds with the latter.

Copper is also abundant in the host's liver. Determinations of copper content of parasites revealed a wide variation (Bremner, 1961) (Table 8). For the liver fluke it ranges from 1·4 to 4·2 μg per worm, i.e. between 77 to 147 ppm of dry weight. It is very interesting that helminths living in the intestinal contents of cattle have only 2–40 ppm of copper; those feeding on the host's

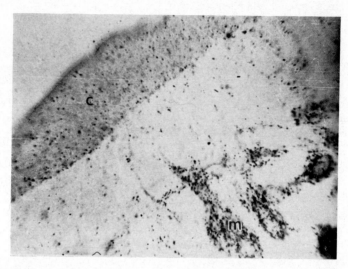

FIG. 53.   Vitamin   C — positive   reaction   to   silver   nitrate   in myoblasts and cuticle (Pantelouris and Hale, 1962).   *m,* myoblasts. *c,* cuticle.

intestinal mucosa have 12–123 ppm, and the blood feeders may have 38–600 ppm. This demonstrates that the copper content of the parasite has no relation to its own copper requirements and must create a metabolic problem of disposal of the excess, i.e. a problem similar to that of iron. In the case of the liver fluke, the presence of copper is probably due to a large extent to the polyphenol oxidase of the yolk glands and eggs; and is also high in *Clonorchis sinensis* reaching 38 mg/100 g of dry tissue (Ma, 1963).

Metabolic Role of the Tegument

Unlike Cestodes, the Trematodes retain a gut, but it is conceivable that they may also make some use of the tegument for obtaining from the medium, or for excreting into it, various products of metabolism. Recent findings (described in other chapters), to the effect that the "cuticle" is in fact a differentiated layer of cytoplasm connected by strands to nucleated living cell bodies constitute circumstantial evidence to this effect.

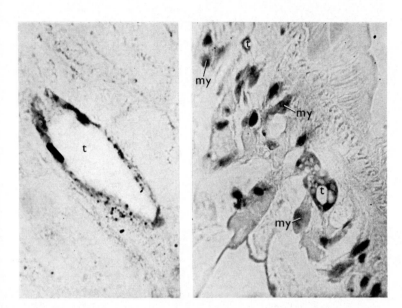

FIG. 54. Left: transverse section through an excretory tubule showing the positive Prussian blue reaction for iron as (blue) rods and dots in the cells of the tubule wall.

Right: the same positive reaction in excretory tubules, *t*, cut transversely and in myoblasts, *my*. (Pantelouris and Hale, 1962).

There is also some more direct evidence. Firstly, Stephenson (1947a), and in more detail, Rohrbacher (1957) and Mansour (1958, 1959) have demonstrated that the addition of fructose or glucose to saline media extends the survival in them of adult liver flukes. This does not seem to be an osmotic effect, as galactose, ribose, maltose, lactose, sucrose and sorbitol are ineffective. The conclusion was that the sugars are used as nutrients; and as their effect remains if the oral suckers of the worms are ligated, it follows that they must enter through the external body surface.

Secondly, the enzyme, alkaline phosphatase, which may be involved in absorption processes, is present in the cuticle of the adult liver fluke as well as in the body wall of the sporocysts (Yamao and Saito, 1952; cited by Bryant and Williams, 1962).

Thirdly, Pantelouris and Gresson (1960) and Pantelouris and Hale (1962) have shown that iron injected in excess into the gut

TABLE 8. COPPER CONTENT OF SOME ADULT HELMINTH PARASITES OF THE COW (FROM BREMNER, 1961)

Parasite	ppm dry weight	μg per worm	Habitat
Nematoda			
Haemonchus placei	146–604	0·028–0·081	calf, abomasum
Ostertagia ostertagi	397	0·005	calf, abomasum
Bunostomum phlebotomum	12–13	0·007–0·008	calf, duodenum
Oesophagostomum radiatum	16–84	0·007–0·043	calf, colon
Trichuris ovis	123	0·10	calf, caecum
Trematoda			
Fasciola hepatica	77–147	1·40–4·20	cow, bile duct
Calicophoron calicophorum	14–26	0·190–0·310	cow, reticulun
Cestoda			
Moniezia benedeni (immature proglottids)	3–7		cow, small intestine
Moniezia benedeni (mature proglottids)	2–5		cow, small intestine
Moniezia expansa	4		cow, small intestine

of the worm appears soon in the cuticle as well as in the cell clusters to which we now know the "cuticle" to be connected. The possibility of the tegument acting as a transport surface was thus raised.

Fourthly, tests with metabolites other than carbohydrates are now in progress. Recently Kureleč and Ehrlich (1963) confirmed that aminoacids are excreted through the tegument. The amount of aminoacids released by the fluke in the medium is reduced by only 6 per cent by the ligation of both the oral sucker and the excretory opening. Furthermore, the aminoacids were shown to enter the parasite from the medium through the tegument.

Similar studies *in vitro* on the uptake of aminoacids from the medium have clarified the paradox of the absence of methionine from liver fluke proteins, reported by Dougherty (1952) and Maekawa and Kushibe (1956); methionine is, however, detected as methionine sulfoxide in chromatograms of whole homogenates (Thorsell and Lienert, 1963). Methionine labelled with S_{35} was added to the medium in which flukes were kept at 37°C for 3 hr. In autoradiographs obtained from sections of such material there was a very high concentration of activity in the cells of the gut epithelium; and a sizeable concentration around and over the testes. When methionine labelled with C_{14} in the methyl group was used there was again a high activity in the gut cells, but over the parenchyma and other tissues activity was low and more or less uniform. These findings were taken to indicate that methionine does become absorbed by the gut cells, but is not incorporated in protein of inner tissues; instead, it is broken down, the sulphur and the methyl group proceeding on different pathways. For comparison, the sulphur from labelled inorganic sulfate accumulated mainly in the vitelline glands. It would appear that sulphur finds its way into mucopolysaccharides of the reticulin network, and also in polyphenols of the yolk, whilst the methyl group is used in other tissues (Pantelouris, 1964a and c).

The evidence for secretion of iron and absorption of amino-acids and sugars through the tegument has naturally led workers to consider the possibility of larger molecules following the same route. Björkman and Thorsell (1964) could detect in the tegument and muscle layers ferritin supplied in the medium *in vitro*; the electron microscope reveals this protein by virtue of a characteristic regular arrangement of ferritin granules. In contrast, Rijaveč *et al.* (1962) failed to detect any absorption of radioiodinated albumin through the tegument.

A different approach was adopted by Pantelouris (1964b). He added insulin to the medium in which flukes were kept for a period of 3 hr. Sections of this and of control material (from medium without the insulin) were stained for glycogen with the Periodic Acid Schiff reagent. It was found that insulin had virtually eliminated the glycogen from the parenchyma, the peripheral muscle layers and the tegument, where glycogen occurs in the form of fine vertical threads. The glycogen of the vitelline glands, on the other hand, was intact, as it in fact remains also in worms subjected to prolonged starvation.

One implication drawn from the effect of insulin was that this protein of relatively low molecular weight reaches the fluke tissues through the tegument.

It appears therefore that some proteins at least — namely ferritin and insulin — as well as smaller molecules (aminoacids and sugars), may be absorbed or secreted through the body surface of the worm. The evidence for this process, however, requires further amplification before conclusions can be drawn concerning its actual role in the nutrition of the parasite.

Effects of Host Hormones

The case of insulin is of interest in another context also, in that a host hormone influences the metabolism of the internal parasite. There is evidence that such effects extend to the uptake of galactose-1-C_{14}, which is reduced by 50 per cent in the presence of insulin.

Furthermore, galactose uptake is similarly affected by yet another hormone, adrenaline (Pantelouris, 1964d). Adrenaline effects on muscular activity of the deganglionated liver fluke preparation have been described in the chapter on the nervous system.

Serotonin also emerges from a series of studies (Mansour *et al.*, 1960; Mansour and Mansour, 1962; Mansour, 1962) as another factor regulating carbohydrate metabolism of the liver fluke. As already noted, it stimulates glycolysis. It has been established that serotonin activates the enzyme, phosphofructokinase, responsible for the transfer of a second phosphate from ATP to fructose-6-phosphate. On closer investigation, serotonin was found primarily to increase the production of adenosine-3, 5-phosphate, this in turn being directly responsible for accelerating glycolysis and glycogenolysis.

Histamine also has been found in liver fluke tissue, at a concentration of 5·2 $\mu g/g$ compared to 7·6μg in the host liver (Mettrick and Telford, 1963. See Pautrizel *et al.*, 1949).

These findings raise the interesting question of metabolic adaptations of the parasite to the hormonal environment in the host, and of the possible importance of such adaptations in determining host-parasite specificity.

Enzymes of Whole Tissue Extracts

It is surprising that we have no detailed enzyme-histochemical study of the gut epithelium, so that we do not yet know what digestive enzymes the liver fluke possesses. The only study of this nature is by Saito (1961) and concerns alkaline and acid phosphatase and lipase. There is, however, an older study, by Pennoit-de Cooman and van Grembergen (1942), of a large number of enzymes, including hydrolytic ones, found in extracts from whole homogenates of the liver fluke, *Planaria* and *Taenia*. Published as it was in Flemish during the war, this paper appears to have been widely overlooked.

Lipases

Tributyrin was used as the substrate. Liberated carboxyl groups were estimated by measuring manometrically the carbon dioxide released from the bicarbonate buffer. Liver fluke, and even more so *Taenia* extracts, had very small activities, in contrast to the free-living *Planaria*. In terms of mm CO_2 released per hr per gram of tissue, measurements were of the order of 600 for *Fasciola* and 300 for *Taenia*, but reached 11,000 to 40,000 for *Planaria*. In his histochemical study Saito, on the other hand, could detect no lipase in the gut epithelium of the liver fluke by Gomori's Tween method.

Cholinesterase

In contrast to *Planaria*, *Taenia* and even more so *Fasciola* were found to possess very little of this enzyme.

Phosphatases

The substrate was β-sodium-glycerophosphate. After incubation with the tissue extract the amount of free inorganic phosphate was estimated. The tests were repeated over a range of pH. Liver fluke phosphatases showed one optimum around pH 4·8, were not inhibited by Mg^{++}, but were inhibited by NaF. For *Taenia* the optimum was between pH 7 and 8. *Planaria*, on the other hand, had two optima, at pH 4·5 and pH 9.

Saito's histochemical reactions, limited to the gut epithelium, were positive for acid phosphatase with a variety of esters as substrates; it was also positive for alkaline phosphatase acting on ATP and fructose-1,6-diphosphate only.

Proteinases

Casein was used as substrate and the carboxyl groups freed were estimated by alkalimetric titration. Whilst the *Fasciola* extracts possessed strong activity at pH 3·6–4·8, they were inactive above or below that range. *Planaria* extract was active at all three parts of the range.

Dipeptidases

These were assayed on glycylglycine with subsequent alkalimetric titration. The level of activity for all three species was more or less comparable to that in mammalian tissues.

Amylase

The liver fluke extract by far exceeded *Planaria* and *Taenia* in amylolytic power. The following amounts of maltose (in grams) were released from potato starch by extracts representing 1 g of tissue: *Planaria* 13–72; *Taenia* 30–92; *Fasciola* 101–210.

Dehydrogenases

Substrates used included succinate, maleate, lactate, α-glycerophosphate, and glutamate. All extracts showed substantial activity, especially with succinate. Only *Planaria* showed some activity with citrate and acetate also.

Catalase

Catalase activity was assayed manometrically. *Fasciola* extracts were roughly five times more potent than *Taenia*, but about 30 times less active than *Planaria* extracts.

Peroxidase

Doubtful reactions, except for the pronounced pseudoperoxidase activity of liver fluke extracts.

Xanthine oxidase

This could not be detected by the methylene blue manometric method.

PART III

PATHOLOGY, CHEMOTHERAPY AND IMMUNOLOGY

CHAPTER 12

THE INVASION OF THE MAMMALIAN HOST

STUDIES on the pathology of fascioliasis have centred around the route taken by the young fluke to reach the liver of the host, the histopathological changes in the liver and bile ducts, the general effects of the disease on the host and its association with other bacterial infections.

The Route to the Liver

Leuckart was inclined to the idea that the young fluke (meta-cercarium) after emerging from the cyst in the host gut and boring its way through the gut wall, is taken up by the blood stream and reaches the liver via the portal vein. Another view advanced by early workers was that the fluke proceeds to the liver through the bile ducts. Again other workers assumed that the fluke travels in the lymph ducts, as flukes are often found in mesenteric lymph nodes. The early work is discussed by Schumacher (1938), and will not be reviewed here.

Newer observations have shown that no flukes can be found in the blood stream and that the bile ducts remain unaffected for some time following an experimental infection. Ssinitzin (1914) and later Shirai (1927) carried out detailed investigations of the events that follow experimental infection. The former, opened the body cavity following infection with cysts given by mouth, and found the flukes crawling on the viscera from 1–2 hr to about 1–2 weeks after the infection. Shirai, using rabbits and guinea pigs, failed to find any parasites in the liver before the 64th day from infection. He fed two guinea pigs for several days with 100 cysts each daily and killed them 20 hr after the last infection. He found the portal vein as well as the vessels of the gut free of flukes; in the liver, he found many worms in the parenchyma but only one within a blood vessel. Histological sections of the gut showed worms in the actual process of burrowing. Shaw (1932) injected a number of cysts into the peritoneum of goats and sheep, and was able to recover liver flukes from the liver. Krull and Jackson (1943) have also produced evidence in support of the peritoneal route hypothesis.

Working on guinea pigs, Schumacher (1956) established that the liver is reached after about two weeks and the bile ducts after about seven weeks from infection. On the surface and in the tissue of the liver the points of penetration are marked by fibrotic changes, and the same route is sometimes used by more than one fluke. Urquhart (1956) described (in rabbits) patches of fibrin on the liver surface, adhesions of the viscera, pale necrotic areas and tracts in the tissue, within 3–7 weeks from infection. As early as 5 weeks after infection some flukes may reach the bile ducts, and after 8 weeks they are all there. Sogoyan (1955, 1956 a and b) and Noguchi (1953) worked with sheep. Intestinal haemorrhages and enlargement may appear within 2–3 days from experimental infection with cysts. Sogoyan believed that in addition to the usual route via the body cavity, some flukes may circulate through lymph and blood vessels, but he observed that any larvae reaching the lungs fail to develop. The liver is entered 6–8 weeks after the infection.

Ectopic Localization

Whilst the liver is the typical tissue sought by the young liver fluke, numerous instances are known of the parasite establishing itself and growing in other locations in the mammalian body. Incidentally, such cases cannot be detected by the demonstration of eggs in the faeces

The most usual place is the lung and the presence of flukes there has been recorded as the cause of acute pneumonia and peribronchial inflammation in sheep (Mychlis, 1959) and cattle (Catellani, 1952; Kochnev, 1950).

The parasite has also been found in lymph nodules (Dziekonski, 1947), and even in the uterus of cattle, causing sterility and endometritis (Thom, 1956 — 4 cases). It is conceivable that in this way the young flukes may even come to settle in the foetus *in utero*. The possibility of pre-natal infection was suggested by

Raillet *et al.* (1913) and confirmed by Bugge (1935). Enigk and Duwel (1959) found liver flukes in 50 out of 661 calves aged under 3 months. Although post-natal infection at that age is not expected normally, it cannot be excluded in principle.

Histopathological Changes

The histopathology of the liver in fascioliasis has been studied by a number of workers. Marek (1927), Turner (1930) and Sogoyan (1955; 1956 a and b) have worked on sheep; Ross and McKay (1929), Bonciu *et al.* (1954) and Lagrange and Gutman (1961) on the guinea pig; Ross and McKay (1926), Urquhart (1956) and Kimura (1961 a and b) on the rabbit; Morrill and Shaw (1942) on cattle; Dawes (1961 a and b; 1962 a and b) on the mouse. These investigations, together with incidental observations recorded in papers dealing with other aspects of the liver fluke disease, provide a clear picture of hepatic changes arising from fascioliasis, and of marked specific differences as to the severity of these changes.

The entry of the metacercaria into the liver tissue ushers in a condition of acute traumatic hepatitis, the severity of which depends on the number of parasites involved. These are now growing fast and devouring the hepatic parenchyma; they form a long somewhat twisting burrow which becomes wider as the size of the parasite increases. Dawes found in the mouse liver that on entry the fluke is 0·3 mm long but it grows to six times that in about 11 days, leaving debris in its wake in the burrow. Leucocytes accumulate and granulation tissue forms; this becomes further collagenized and finally the tracts become filled with fibrous tissue, taking on the appearance of necrotic tracts. Portal vessels near the tracts become oedematous and large numbers of lymphocytes collect around them. Also the smaller bile ducts become hyperplastic (Figs. 55–56). Patches of black pigments appear, due to the haematin discharged by the fluke (Campbell, 1961). It is probable that the liver parenchyma recovers in view of the powers of regeneration possessed by liver tissue (at least in cattle, Morrill and Shaw, 1942).

The aftermaths of this stage include patches of fibrin on the liver surface, adhesions between liver and other viscera, fibrous

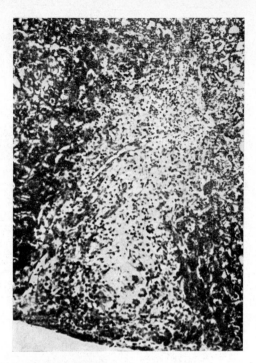

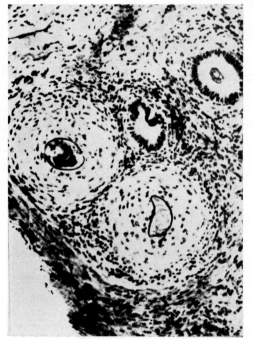

Fig. 55. Top: A small fluke tract below the surface of a rabbit's liver, freshly healed. It is filled with loose connective tissue interspersed with phagocytes, degenerating multinucleated liver giant cells and a few young bile ducts (Urquhart, 1956).

Bottom: Granulomata forming around eggs released in the liver tissue by flukes in experimentally infected rabbits (Urquhart, 1956).

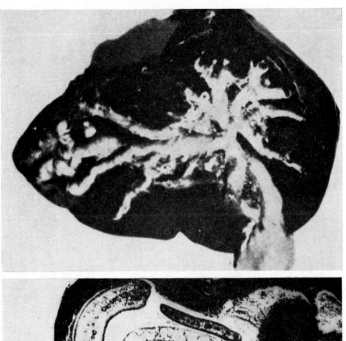

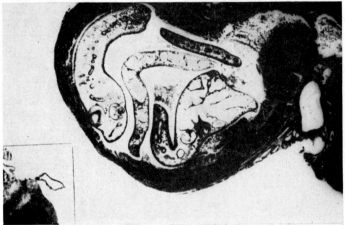

FIG. 56.   Top: Photograph of an infected liver to show the distention and calcification of the bile ducts (Morrill, 1942).

Bottom: Transverse section through a distended and thickened bile duct of the rabbit and of several liver flukes contained therein. Insert: normal width of a corresponding duct (Urquhart, 1956).

layers on the peritoneal surface and adhesions between viscera, also granulomata around eggs or even occasionally around adult flukes.

As the flukes leave the liver for the bile ducts, the acute stage gives way to a chronic stage. The smaller bile ducts may become obstructed by fluke eggs, others become enlarged and their epithelium is damaged; eggs infiltrating the duct wall cause granulomata and accumulations of macrophages and fibroblasts. The bile ducts may also rupture in places. According to Morrill and Shaw, the walls of the bile ducts react with epithelial hyperplasia, and the calcification of ducts may have a protective significance.

In summary, Urquhart described the clinical syndrome of hepatic fascioliasis as a coarse cirrhosis, caused by: (1) the healing migration tracts, (2) infarcts, (3) chronic cholangitis from adult flukes in the larger bile ducts, (4) hyperplasia of connective tissue and biliary elements in the portal tracts, and (5) granulomata round eggs seeded in tissues.

Bugge (1927c) disputes whether the sheep bile ducts are ever calcified as a result of liver fluke infection. Discussing ectopic localization in the lungs (Bugge, 1927c) the same author describes the gradual growth of the nodes containing the flukes. Soon after the cercaria reach the lungs, the nodes are pea-size and containing the youngest flukes with unbranched gut. Later they may become filled with a brown-red fluid, and surrounded by connective tissue; the flukes now are about 3–10 mm long. Finally the nodes in the lung tissue may reach the size of a nut and become encapsulated and are found to contain adult or dead flukes.

Effect on Meat

Not only is there liver damage, but the meat of infected animals seems to be of poorer quality, darker in colour and to contain more volatile fatty acids than that of healthy animals, according to Goncharuk (1959 a and b); this author based his conclusions on the examination of forty-four infected and eighteen healthy carcasses of cattle. Regarding quantity, he found that the infected animals produced 30 per cent less meat than the healthy animals (Fig. 57, from Sinclair, 1962). Vasilev (1961) compared meat samples

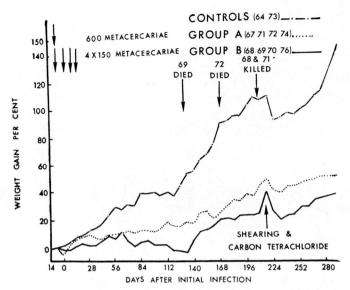

FIG. 57. Graph from Sinclair (1962) to show the effect on weight gain of sheep of infection with 600 metacercaria in one dose (group A), or with four doses of 150 metacercaria each at intervals of a week (group B). Uninfected controls.

from one healthy calf and four that were infected for 8·5 months. In the latter, fat content was severely reduced but water content increased; the pH index was also higher.

Variation in Susceptibility

The pathological changes brought about by fascioliasis differ markedly with species.

In the pig the lesions seem to be lighter and to consist mainly in encapsulation of parasites and distention and hardening of the bile ducts (Frenkel, 1907; Gebauer, 1958).

Some observations on the horse were made by Ugrin and Skovronski (1959), following an outbreak of fascioliasis in animals grazed alongside cattle in the Lvov region. Of seventy-four adult horses, a quarter were found infected, and of twelve foals, half had the infection. It was noted that even with hundreds of flukes in the bile ducts, the livers were free of cirrhosis and were not enlarged.

Among laboratory animals, the survival rate after equivalent infection was found to be 65·5 per cent for albino rats, 6·6 per cent for Syrian hamsters and 13·2 per cent for cotton rats. Also the rats were found to carry significantly fewer flukes than the rabbits (Lämmler, 1959).

Other instances of species differences in susceptibility are given in p. 16 in connexion with *Fascioloides* infections, and on p. 131 for infections with *F. gigantica*.

It is also probable that even within species there are differences in this respect from strain to strain. Shaw (1946) remarked that in Oregon, local cattle show milder symptoms of infection, and become infected less easily, than the zebu hybrids raised in the same area.

Frenkel (1907) and Bugge and Müller (1928) find that the liver fluke fails to mature in the pig, where it is effectively encapsulated and calcified.

Comparison with F. gigantica Infections

In his experiments already mentioned, Sogoyan infected sheep with cysts of both *Fasciola hepatica* and *F. gigantica,* and thus was able to compare the damage to the liver caused by the two species. The latter species reaches the liver within 10–11 weeks after the infection as against 6–8 weeks for *F. hepatica,* and stays there much longer; on occasion it was found in the liver 18 whole weeks after infection.

In *F. gigantica* infections, Sogoyan recorded alterations in parenchymatous organs other than the liver and attributed them to toxins; these alterations include: in the heart, swelling of capillaries and haematomas under the pericardium, appearing from the 20th day after infection onwards; in the spleen, hyperaemia and enlargement of the pulp during the acute stage of the disease; and in the kidneys, progressive glomerulonephritis.

Further comparative studies were carried out by Davtyan (1953, 1956). Sheep experimentally infected with *Fasciola gigantica* died within 51–109 days; the immediate cause of death being severe haemorrhages from the liver into the intraperitoneal cavity. Maturity is reached within 94–107 days. Sheep treated with hexachlorethane or carbon tetrachloride died when the treatment was given in three doses on the 38th, 40th and 42nd days of infection, but survived when it was postponed until the 68th, 70th and 72nd days.

In another experiment, sheep were given either 250–300 cercaria of *F. gigantica,* or 300–1000 cercaria of *F. hepatica.* Although the first group carried 33–265 flukes in the liver and the others 122–870, the latter survived and reached the chronic stage of fascioliasis whilst the first all died.

When the test was repeated with bovines, the results were reversed. It would seem therefore, in Davtyan's view, that *F. gigantica* is a parasite specifically adapted to bovine hosts.

Toxic Effects

To the direct damage caused in the liver tissue, there should be added the effects of toxins released in the host's circulation.

As early as 1906 it was noted that a filtered aqueous extract of liver fluke tissue is poisonous to rabbits; if injected intraperitoneally it kills the rabbit within 3 days, but it becomes nonpoisonous if it is first heated to 50–60°C (Albanese, 1906 — quoted by Weinland and Brand, 1926).

Experimental injection of liver fluke extracts in animals causes marked eosinophilia and indeed the latter is a constant symptom in fascioliasis. Other toxic and anaphylactic accidents may also occur (Marcheboeuf and Mandoul, 1939 a and b). Blood of infected animals was found to haemolyze blood cells of other animals of the same or other species (Guerrini, 1908).

Pautrizel (1951) attributed effects of this kind to a fraction of fluke tissue that can be obtained by precipitation with warm ethyl alcohol from the trichloracetic acid extract. He described it as a glucide-lipido-polypeptide complex.

Deschiens and Poirier (1950, 1953) compared extracts prepared in three different ways: (a) Isotonic aquatic extract of liver fluke tissue corresponding to 0·8 g of tissue/ml of extracting medium. This was given by injection to three guinea pigs, at the rate of one injection (1 ml/kg body weight) every other day for 16 days. Whilst before injection the blood eosinophils in these three animals were 2%, 2% and 0%, they rose to 14%, 12% and 12% afterwards. The initial normal myelograms of 7–9% rose to 15%, 20% and 20%. Biopsy showed alveolar stasis and oedema in the lungs, vein stasis and pycnosis of nuclei in the liver, and irritative lesions of the convoluted tubules and glomeruli of the kidney. (b) An isotonic trichloracetic acid extract. Injected for 32 days, this extract raised eosinophil counts of 1%, 1% and 1% to 9%, 6% and 7%, and myelograms from normal to 15–16%. When the animals were killed, the lungs showed serious oedema, desquamation and exudation of the bronchs; the liver, steatosis, stasis and diffuse infiltration; the kidneys, haemorrhagic oedema, glomerular dilatation, tumofaction of the tubular epithelium, and necrosis of the convoluted tubules. (c) the third type of extract (glucides, lipids and polypeptides) was obtained from the trichloracetic acid extract by precipitation with alcohol and dispersal in saline. Eosinophilia again rose to 5%, 12%, 12% and 14% in four guinea pigs and the myelogram to 12–22%. The lungs showed alveolitis and atelectasia by capillary dilation; the liver, steatosis and oedema near the portal veins; the kidney, necrosis of convoluted tubules.

In summary, eosinophilia was worst with the aquatic and mildest with the trichloracetic acid extract. However, the other lesions were mildest with the aquatic, more severe with the polypeptide and worst with the trichloracetic acid extracts.

Serious necrosis of the adrenal glands was diagnosed in guinea pigs injected with liver fluke extract (Poirier and Deschiens, 1961), and the vitamin C content of the adrenals was found lowered in cases where the cirrhosis was severe (Zioto, 1960). Further toxic effects on the spleen, kidneys, heart and brain have been described by Sogoyan (1958) in the case of sheep carrying the parasite.

Other Symptoms

A variety of symptoms follow the presence of liver fluke in the tissues of the mammalian host.

Noguchi et al. (1958) carried out various tests of liver function and other examinations on 4 sheep given metacercaria and on 2 controls. The infected animals stopped putting on weight after about 5 weeks, but resumed after about 90 days from the time of infection. The suspension of growth would therefore roughly coincide with the acute stage of fascioliasis, when the flukes are feeding on the liver. After the 13th week from infection the level of bilirubin in the serum and of urobilinogen in the urine rose above normal. Also, from the 9th week onwards, the number of red cells and the ratio of albumin to globulin fell. Other tests, including prothrombin-time and blood-sugar estimations, revealed no clear-cut differences between controls and infected animals.

The alkaline phosphatase level remains normal and there is no bilirubinemia, hence the flow of bile is not, in the view of Urquhart, obstructed. He checked this point by a bromsulphalein excretion test and confirmed that excretion of this compound does not differ in normal and control rabbits; it does rise however if the bile ducts are experimentally ligated. Ehrlich *et al.* (1960 a and b) detected (in cattle) a slight but constant rise of bilirubin level in the blood.

An increase of globulins in the blood plasma, as in so many infections, was detected by Kona, 1957; Maglajic *et al.*, 1959; Ehrlich *et al.* (1960), whilst Deschiens and Bénex (1960 a and b) were able to distinguish the plasma protein pattern of (human) cases of fascioliasis from that of unaffected controls but not from cases carrying another parasite, *Schistosoma*. The peritoneal exudate shows the same composition as the plasma (Kona, 1957 a and b).

The blood iron, phosphorus, magnesium, sugar and potassium levels may all fall, the calcium level being only slightly affected (Ibrovic and Gall-Palla, 1959; Ugrin and Skovronski, 1959; Sinclair, 1960).

Describing the progress of the disease in rabbits, Kimura (1961 a and b) distinguished three stages: Firstly, in the period of up to 50 days after infection, there is severe oligocythemia, anaemia, raised temperature, leucocytosis and eosinophilia. These symptoms are followed by a period of aggravated oligocythemia and anaemia, diarrhoea, swelling of the face etc. Oligocythemia and hypochromia also characterise the period after the 200th day from the time of infection.

A reduction of erythropoietic activity in the bone marrow, coupled with increased leucopoiesis, was demonstrated (in buffaloes) (Giordano, 1959).

The course of symptoms in sheep was followed systematically by Sinclair (1962) for nine months after an experimental infection. The increase in γ-globulin is followed in time by a progressive fall of the albumin level in the serum. Whilst the number of red cells falls, in all probability due to loss of blood especially as the flukes reach the adult stage, their replenishment is prevented by some toxic factor acting on the bone marrow hemopoietic tissue. The fall of magnesium and calcium levels of the blood may roughly be put at a maximum of 25 per cent; removal of adult flukes by treatment with carbon tetrachloride permits the levels of these two elements to return gradually towards the normal. The values obtained in tests on two sheep just before they died of the chronic phase of the disease, together with those from a control animal, are given in Table 9.

Typical and severe symptoms affecting the nervous system have been described by Muravev (1950). "Fine-wool" sheep in the Dniepropetrovsk area were so affected by excessive infestation that they became restless to begin with, hitting their heads against walls, etc. This stage was followed by one of inertia, the animals standing or lying motionless without eating; they died within about a week from exhaustion. Temperature remained normal throughout but the mucous membranes became yellow and the

TABLE 9. BIOCHEMICAL ESTIMATIONS ON SAMPLES TAKEN IMMEDIATELY BEFORE DEATH FROM TWO SHEEP WITH CHRONIC FASCIOLIASIS (SINCLAIR, 1962)

Estimation	Sheep 69	Sheep 72	Control
Erythrocytes (10^6/mm^3)	1·4	5·2	10·2
Haemoglobin (g/100 ml)	2·1	3·9	10·3
Packed cell volume (per cent)	6·0	13·5	30·5
Leucocytes (10^3/mm^3)	15·7	5·8	7·4
Serum calcium (mg/100 ml)	9·1	9·1	10·9
Serum magnesium (mg/100 ml)	1·8	1·7	2·4
Total serum protein (g/100 ml)	2·6	4·4	5·9
Albumin	1·1	1·3	3·8
a_1 Globulin	0·2	0·4	0·3
a_2 Globulin	0·4	0·8	0·55
β Globulin	0·3	0·5	0·35
γ Globulin	0·6	1·4	0·9
Fluke eggs/g faeces	4000	2400	0
Flukes recovered at post mortem	188	221	0

Note: Sheep No. 69 was infected with 600 metacercaria in one dose; sheep No. 72 was given the same number of metacercaria in four equal weekly doses.

wool started falling off. At post-mortem, liver and gall bladder were greatly enlarged, the liver often to twice its normal size. Several hundreds of *Fasciola hepatica* were crowding the bile ducts, but generally no other parasites were found — except Echinococci in some cases.

It is claimed by Goryanova (1957) that the presence of the liver fluke affects the nervous system in such a way as to modify the frequency and strength of contraction of the rumen wall; and that such effects can be detected even in cases where other symptoms are not yet obvious. She describes tests in which animals were given pre-digested cud after a fast of about 10 hr and the rumen contractions in response to this stimulus were recorded by ruminograph. The recording shows in comparison to healthy animals, a weakening of rumen contractions which persists for about $2\frac{1}{2}$ months even after treatment with hexachlorethane. Unfortunately, Goryanova's paper gives no illustration of recordings from affected and healthy animals.

CHAPTER 13

FASCIOLIASIS AND BACTERIAL
INFECTIONS

It is to be expected that, in its migration through the host tissues, the young liver fluke may introduce bacteria from the gut. Furthermore, the damage it causes to the liver results in the flareup of certain bacteria that are present but normally remain latent in that organ.

Bile from over 700 cattle slaughtered in abattoirs was collected in the Netherlands and examined for paratyphoid or other bacteria. The samples from 614 Dutch cattle were contaminated in 39 per cent of the cases, from 48 Irish in 47 per cent of cases and from 64 Danish cattle in 7 per cent. The high incidence in the Dutch and Irish cattle was attributed to the frequency of fascioliasis in them (Gunst and Manen, 1948).

Workers at Munich have also demonstrated that 1·2–1·6 per cent of cattle parasitized with liver fluke are carriers of the Gärtner bacillus (*Salmonella enteritides*) (Glässer and Weitzner, 1948). Similarly, parasitized sheep seem to harbour *Bacterium coli* in the duodenum and gall bladder, whilst in healthy animals, the bacterium is restricted to the lower ends of the gut (Haberkern, 1951; Schindler, 1951; von Krudener, 1952).

Clostridium welchii type A was found to be abundant in animals suffering from fascioliasis during an epidemic in Yugoslavia (Butozan et al., 1961). Fascioliasis was also found to be associated, with tuberculosis infection of the affected livers (Keller, 1952).

A special case of bacterial infection accompanying fascioliasis is that of the notorious "black disease" of sheep.

This disease was first reported from New South Wales in 1895, and was initially described as "braxy" by a mistaken analogy to the disease known in Britain under this name.

The affected animals showed no striking external symptoms,

except that they were drowsy, lagged behind, and found it progressively more difficult to catch up with the others. Respiration became shallow and of the Cheynes–Stokes type. Death supervened suddenly and without struggle.

Dodd (1918, 1921) carried out a large number of post-mortems and was also able to produce the disease experimentally by injecting blood or fluid from diseased into healthy animals. Two types of bacilli, one resembling the causative agent for braxy, and the other the agent for malignant oedema, were found in the fluids; but feeding of such bacilli or of infected tissues failed to cause the disease. Eventually, this worker discovered that the bacteria found in the blood at post-mortems were not in the blood in autopsies; it followed that they must be hidden in some organ during life. In fact, the liver of the diseased animals showed areas of coagulative necrosis with zones of leucocytes surrounding them and masses of a bacillus between the two. This bacillus was filamentous, gram-positive and anaerobic.

Dodd commented that the conditions favouring black disease are the same as those favouring fascioliasis and speculated that, in its migration through the liver, the fluke might be introducing the bacterial infection.

Albiston (1927) found similarities between the bacterium present in black disease and *B. oedematiens*. In the 1930's Turner (1928, 1930 a and b) resumed the study of the disease and confirmed Dodd's description of the necrotic lesions. More important, he associated the disease more closely with infection of the necrotic area by *Bacillus oedematiens*, occasionally accompanied by other anaerobes. Not only the liver fluke but also another migratory parasitic helminth, *Cysticercus pisiformis*, or even damage of the liver with carbon tetrachloride, can usher in the disease, according to his findings.

To study the route of entry of the bacillus, Turner injected inactivated spores of the bacillus intratracheally and discovered that they are taken up by endothelial phagocytes. In stained preparations up to 30 spores can be seen in one phagocyte. Later the spores seem to accumulate in organs where circulation is slowed down, i.e. the liver and the bone marrow (Table 10).

Turner argued that this might be the way in which live spores

K

TABLE 10. INJECTION OF TOXIN-FREE SPORES OF *Bacillus oedematiens* BY VARIOUS ROUTES (TURNER, 1930)

Route	Animal	Dose (in Millions)	Result
Subcutaneous	Guinea-pig	50	Innocuous up to 9 months
	Sheep	2×50	Innocuous up to 9 months
Intramuscular	Guinea-pig	$2\frac{1}{2} + 5$	Innocuous up to 9 months
	Rabbits	50	Innocuous up to 3 months
	Sheep	2×50	Innocuous up to 9 months
Intraperitoneal	Guinea-pig	$2\frac{1}{2} + 5$	Innocuous up to 9 months
		25	Innocuous up to 4 months
	Sheep	2×50	Innocuous up to 9 months
Intrapleural	Guinea-pig	$2\frac{1}{2} + 5$	Innocuous up to 9 months
Intratracheal	Rabbit	50	Innocuous up to 12 months
	Sheep	2×50	Innocuous up to 9 months
Intrahepatic	Rabbit	$12\frac{1}{2}$	Innocuous up to 3 months
Intratesticular	Guinea-pig	5	Only a short test, 19–22$\frac{1}{2}$ hr
Feeding	Rabbits, Sheep	Undetermined	Innocuous up to 5 months at least
	Guinea-pig	$2\frac{1}{2} + 5$	70% innocuous, 30% died
Intravenous	Rabbit (a)	England — 50	Innocuous up to 19 days at least
	Rabbit (b)	Australia — $2\frac{1}{2}$ to 50	All died
	Sheep	2×50	Innocuous up to 9 months

are reaching the liver naturally, i.e. by being taken up by phago-cytes of the pharyngeal lymph glands. The spores are toxin-free and they would presumably remain latent in the liver in the absence of liver fluke infection. (The same micro-organism was also found in 3 out of 18 rabbits and in 1 out of 10 crows examined.)

Turner's theory was soon vindicated by workers in Scotland. *Bacillus* (or *Clostridium*) *oedematiens* was found present in a latent state in about a third of healthy sheep livers in areas where "watery braxy" (as the disease is called locally) is endemic. The spores become activated as the migrating liver flukes destroy liver cells; they then produce toxins which are responsible for the necrosis and for the sudden death within 12–24 hr.

In the Caithness area, black disease was absent from farms on the acid soils disliked by *Limnaea truncatula*, and also from well-drained soils. Outbreaks coincided with the season of cercarial ingestion in autumn (Jamieson *et al.*, 1948; Jamieson, 1949; Jamieson and Thomson, 1949). This constitutes a confirmation of the connexion of the two diseases.

"Black disease" is to be distinguished from "braxy". In the latter, liver-fluke infestation is not always present, the primary lesion is not in the liver but in the abomasum, and hoggs are more affected than adult animals.

In black disease, the skinned fleece shows intensely congested blood vessels and the liver is engorged with blood and necrotic areas. As the blood in the skin of carcasses turns black, this may have been the source of the name "black disease". The pericar-dium is distended with clear fluid which may be the cause of the sudden deaths, by compression of the heart. On dissection the fluid soon coagulates.

The detection of the micro-organism involved and the elucida-tion of the role of the liver fluke, opened the way to methods of control and prevention. As early as 1927 Albiston attempted to produce immunity to black disease. He cultured the bacteria in-volved and injected them live in guinea pigs, rabbits and sheep— with the result that the animals promptly died.

He then used germ-free culture filtrates as antigens but could get no immunity for guinea pigs with the dose he used. He also tested killed bacteria and filtered exudate obtained *post-mortem* from infected sheep. These proved toxic to guinea pigs and provided no immunity. He noted the resemblance of the micro-organism to *B. oedematiens*.

In recent years, Wellcome Laboratories have produced and tested three types of antisera formed by sheep given injections of either a toxoid, an alum precipitate of the toxoid, or formalinized whole culture of the bacterium (Jamieson and Thomson, 1949). The best results were obtained with antisera to the two latter antigens. The toxoid antiserum reduced mortality to one-third of that in a control group of sheep, the anaculture antiserum to one-quarter. Similar encouraging results with the same serum were obtained by Parker (1948).

Two products are now available from the same Laboratories. For prevention, a vaccine to be injected subcutaneously in the summer or early autumn. For immediate protection where the disease appears, an antiserum used to impart immediate passive immunity.

Not only does the liver fluke facilitate the entry of bacteria into the tissues, but the reverse also appears to be true. Infection of guinea pigs with metacercaria accompanied by *Bacillus subtilis* resulted in a much larger number of parasites than normal developing in the animals (Higashi, 1960 a and b). Whilst the infection rate was 75 per cent when the cysts were given without bacteria, it rose to 100 per cent when micro-organisms were also given. Furthermore the average number of parasites found at autopsy was 11–26 as against 3 in controls. Intraperitoneal inflammation, quite severe, was found on dissection.

It might be worth noting that in cattle in Kenya an inverse relationship was observed between the numbers of liver flukes (*F. gigantica*) and of hydatid cysts of *Echinococcus granulosus* (Froyd, 1960).

CHAPTER 14

MAINTENANCE *IN VITRO* AND
PHARMACOLOGICAL TESTS

Maintenance *in Vitro*

As for all internal parasites, a technique for maintaining the liver fluke in good condition *in vitro* is a prerequisite of physiological studies, and of tests for anthelminthic compounds. Whilst earlier workers could maintain the parasite alive in Ringer's saline for up to only 12 hr, Stephenson (1947) was able to double this period by using a saline of pH 9·2 and of the following composition:

NaCl	115 mM
KCl	5 mM
CaCl$_2$	1 mM
borax	8·5 mM.

Further improvement was obtained when a carbohydrate was added as a source of energy. The best result, survival for 72 hr, was obtained by the addition to the saline of 45 mM of fructose. Glucose, galactose or maltose, lactose or sucrose were less efficient in that order. However, the sugars lower the pH, and Stephenson tested the effect of different pH on survival, obtaining the results outlined in Fig. 58. To take these into account, he finally recommended a solution of the same composition as above, but with fructose (or, if this is not available, then glucose) added at the rate of 30 mM. This solution has a pH of 8·6 and gives a survival of 40 hr. Rohrbacher (1957) actually found that survival in this saline can be further extended to 9 days by controlling bacteria with antibiotics.

A further and very important improvement was introduced by Dawes (1954), who criticized Stephenson's technique for: (a) the presence of borax, and (b) the probable bacterial contamination of the flukes at the start of the tests, and their moribund condition. He replaced Stephenson's saline with the Hédon-Fleig solution, and outlined a procedure for obtaining nearly bacteria-free parasites and for maintaining them bacteria-free. His procedure is as follows: The saline is sterilized by passing through a Seitz filter, and the worms are removed aseptically from the liver as

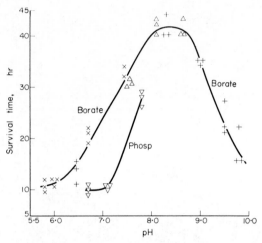

Fig. 58.   The effect of pH on the length of survival of liver flukes in saline according to Stephenson (1947).

freshly as possible. Solutions are renewed several times a day, and even so special precautions must be taken to prevent contamination with air-borne bacteria. Incidentally, if this is achieved, the pH of the solution remains constant, as shown by drops of phenol red included in the saline as an indicator. Nor is the parasite very sensitive to pH changes (Clegg, 1957).

Rohrbacher's approach was different. He also ensured that the flukes were bacteria-free to begin with, and then he used a saline with antibiotics. Tyrode solution allowed longer survival but normal mobility and colour were lost after a week. The addition of aminoacids, cholesterol, or Injection Crude Liver, alone or in combination, had no appreciable effects. However, the addition of Injection Crude Liver together with autoclaved liver extract made a great difference. With the conditions finally adopted, survival of the parasites in good condition for three weeks — and for another week still alive but deteriorating — was obtained

TABLE 11. SURVIVAL OF LIVER FLUKES *in vitro* IN DIFFERENT MEDIA; EXPERIMENT BY ROHRBACHER (1957)

Number of flukes surviving under anaerobic conditions; one fluke per bottle in 50 ml of solution

	0	1	2	3	4	5	6	7	8	9	10	1	2	3	4	5	6	7	8	9	20	1	2	3	4
1. Stephenson's saline, not sterile; flukes transported while still in bile ducts	8	8	8	8	0																				
2. Stephenson's saline, not sterile; flukes removed from bile duct at once	3	3	3	2	0																				
3. Stephenson's saline, sterile	3	3	2	2	2	1	1	1	1	1	0														
4. Rohrbacher's saline	3	3	3	3	3	2	2	2	2	2	2	2	0												
5. Tyrode's solution	11	11	11	11	11	11	11	11	10	9	5	5	3	3	3	2	2	1	1	1	1	1	1	1	0
6. Tyrode's with liver extract	3	3	3	2	2	2	2	2	2	2	2	2	2	2	2	1	1	1	1	1	1	0			
7. Rohrbacher's with liver extract	14	14	13	13	10	8	8	8	5	4	4	3	3	2	2	2	2	2	2	2	2	2	2	2	0
8. Rohrbacher's enriched medium	18	18	18	18	18	17	16	16	16	14	13	13	12	10	9	9	8	8	8	8	8	8	8	8	8

(Table 11). The solutions used by Stephenson, Dawes and Rohrbacher are set out in Table 12.

In all this work, the condition of the parasite was judged by mobility and colour. Clegg however used an additional criterion, the appearance of abnormal morulae in spermatogenesis (see p. 93); this seems to be an index very sensitive to changes in the medium. He found that the Hédon-Fleig medium can be further

TABLE 12. SOLUTIONS FOR THE MAINTENANCE *in vitro* OF ADULT LIVER FLUKES

Amounts given in grams per litre of distilled water.

	Stephenson*	Tyrode†	Hédon-Fleig‡	Rohrbacher¶
NaCl	8·64	8·00	7·00	2·40
KCl	0·745	0·201	0·30	0·75
CaCl$_2$	0·11	0·20	0·10	0·55
MgCl$_2$.6H$_2$O	—	0·10	—	0·20
MgSO$_4$	—	—	0·30	—
NaH$_2$PO$_4$.H$_2$O	—	0·05	—	—
Na$_2$HPO$_4$.2H$_2$O	—	—	0·50	2·70
NaHCO$_3$	—	1·00	—	0·84
Na$_2$ citrate	—	—	—	2·90
Na$_2$B O$_7$.10H$_2$O	2·29	—	—	—
Glucose	5·40	1·00	1·00	3·60
Cholesterol				1·80

* Stephenson's saline: Tested by Stephenson (1947) who obtained survival of up to 24 hr. Rohrbacher (1957), by first sterilising the flukes with antibiotics and by removing them immediately from the slaughtered host, obtained in it a survival of 9 days.

† Tyrode's solution: Rohrbacher obtained in this survival of up to 21 days, but the flukes were in a moribund condition after the first week.

‡ Hédon-Fleig solution: Clegg (1957) with aseptic conditions and using special cellulose culture tubes obtained in this a survival of 10 days or more.

¶ Rohrbacher's saline: Rohrbacher, always using flukes freed of bacteria with antibiotics, obtained in this solution a survival of 12 days and normal movement for 10. Rohrbacher's enriched medium consists of 800 ml of the above saline without the cholesterol plus 200 ml of autoclaved liver extract and 10 ml of Injection Crude Liver. To prepare the liver extract, homogenize cattle liver in an equal volume of distilled water, autoclave to coagulate the protein, filter, bottle and autoclave. The Injection Crude Liver can be obtained commercially (Thompson Inc., Stamford, Conn.)

improved by the addition of an equal volume of horse serum, when only a few abnormal morulae appear after 48 hr.

Rediae can also be maintained *in vitro*. Working with *Fascioloides magna*, Friedl (1961) was able to maintain them in haemolymph of their host-snail *Limnaea stagnalis*, or in Clark's insect tissue culture medium. The haemolymph is the better medium of the two; after autoclaving, it allows the survival of rediae for 13 days. The same author tested the survival of rediae in chemically defined media. Proline, hydroxyproline and serine enhanced survival as compared to un-supplemented saline.

Pharmacological Tests

Whilst media for maintaining the liver fluke *in vitro* for rather long periods are now available, most pharmacological tests so far have been carried out in simple saline, to which the compound tested was added at various concentrations. The effect on length of survival or on muscular activity has been compared to controls kept in saline without the drug. Even the property of stimulating muscular activity of the worm might prove useful, in that it might loosen up the worms from the bile duct and result in their elimination from the host.

To record the muscular activity of liver flukes *in vitro*, the worm is connected by hook and thread to a recording lever. Fresh worms maintain a rhythmic activity in Ringer's solution of pH 6·5–8·5 for at least two hours. (Incidentally, whilst this is the rule for flukes from cattle it is rather unusual with flukes from sheep.) Cessation of movement of the worm due to the paralyzing effect of a drug must be distinguished from a moribund condition. For this purpose 1:5000 amphetamine sulphate or 1:200,000 nicotine is added to the medium; this reverses any paralyzing action and the rhythmic movements are resumed in worms that are not moribund or dead.

Making use of such procedures, Chance and Mansour (1949) tested a number of chemicals, namely chlorinated hydrocarbons, various drugs known to be effective against *Ascaris,* and also umbelliferone, pilleturine, extract felix mas and gentian violet. The liver fluke proved sensitive to some extent to all of these.

The chlorinated hydrocarbons stimulate movement at low concentrations but kill at high. Phenothiazine and also certain drugs lethal to bilharzial worms proved inactive against *Fasciola*.

These authors selected the drugs to test from compounds known for anthelminthic activity. Another group of workers decided to test drugs effective against malaria, on the idea that the liver fluke, whilst still in the liver parenchyma, is in fact in the same environment as the pre-erythrocytic stages of the malarial plasmodia (Sharaf *et al.*, 1960). Atebrin, camoquin and daraprin stimulated movement, although in high concentrations the latter caused paralysis.

Lienert (1949) and Lienert and Mathois (1952 a and b) tested 22 substances selected on the basis that (a) they are eliminated unaltered through the bile and (b) they are less toxic to cattle and sheep than the drugs in use.

The following compounds exhibited efficient action *in vitro* against the liver fluke: quinozol and desoxycholic acid, and to a lesser extent: eosin, fluorescein, sodium iodide, sulfamethazin, Congo red, phenol red.

From another group of 27 compounds, mercurochrom (disodium salt of dibromohydroxymercuri-fluorescein), and to a lesser extent phenyl mercuriacetate and ascorbic acid, proved highly efficient. In the case of these substances, however, it is not known whether or not they are broken down in the host. Breakdown before they reach the bile would of course make them ineffective *in vivo*. Stephenson (1947) noted on the other hand that certain known anthelminthics were innocuous to the liver fluke *in vitro* (gentian violet, ethylene dichloride, carbon tetrachloride) but did not study the question in detail. Certain bacteriostatics (acriflavin, merthiolate, silver proteins) proved toxic to the liver fluke when added to the saline in which Stephenson maintained the parasite *in vitro*.

Piperazine stimulates movement at first, but causes paralysis later (Barke, 1958). In practice, a piperazine preparation ("Distan") proved valueless against the parasite in cattle (Enigk and Duwel, 1958). Epinephrine has no effect because the phenol oxidase present in the tissues of the parasite (p. 100) oxidizes it at a high rate.

Benzothiazoles have been tested, the most potent proving to be 6-nitro-2-mercaptobenzothiazole, which is lethal to the parasite *in vitro* at a concentration of only 1 : 8000 (Mackie *et al.*, 1955). Numerous other compounds have also been tested and extensive screening of other likely chemicals is being carried out by industrial laboratories.

Metacercaria also can be kept in water provided this is regularly renewed (Grigoryan, 1959). "Miracil D" (1 : 20,000), Nile blue and Meldola blue were found to kill these larvae whilst antimony compounds did not (Lagrange and Scheegmans, 1950). The persistence of Nile blue in the host tissue was investigated by injection into mice, and various routes of administration were compared. However, the authors expressed doubts as to the usefulness of Nile blue *in vivo* because, if injected intravenously, it can give rise to thrombosis.

Of course, tests *in vitro* such as described above are only preliminary to studies *in vivo*; only the latter can decide the best means and routes of administering the drug and of achieving an effective concentration of it in the tissues. Furthermore, *in vivo* studies will reveal whether the drug has any side effects on the host or whether it is metabolized by the host to ineffective compounds.

It is not easy in tests *in vivo* to know the number of worms expelled as a result of the drug and the number of those left intact in the host; and egg counts are subject to many factors other than number of parasites. Vodrazka (1963) overcame this difficulty in tests of anthelminthics against the liver fluke in sheep by inserting a tube and a sieve in the main bile duct; the sieve stops the dead flukes for later collection and count, whilst it lets the bile through.

Lienert's "Leberegeltest" consists in the implantation of 6–8 adult flukes under the skin of albino rats of a standard size (about 200 g). Drugs are injected or given orally, and after a few days the flukes are recovered and examined. In untreated rats all flukes are usually found alive. This speedy and inexpensive test is suitable for screening substances expected to reach the flukes through the blood, but is not suitable for substances concentrating in the bile. The value of the test has been confirmed in experiments with hexachloroethane, hexachlorophene, bromochlorophene, bithionol, fluothane and diaphene (Lienert, 1960a, b, c, and d; 1962; 1963a, and b; Lienert and Jahn, 1962a, and b).

CHAPTER 15

ANTHELMINTHICS USED AGAINST THE LIVER FLUKE

Carbon Tetrachloride

Carbon tetrachloride is widely used against the liver fluke and its effectiveness is well proven. However, it exerts toxic effects on the liver of the host (especially on cattle), a fact that imposes restrictions and precautions in its use.

It is sometimes given orally in capsules or in the fluid state, but it is preferable to inject it subcutaneously or intramuscularly, diluted in liquid paraffin or some other oil (Gavrilyuk, 1956).

Effectiveness of Carbon Tetrachloride

This compound cannot act on the young liver flukes as they migrate through the liver (Shaginyan, 1955). As a result, treatment has to be repeated at intervals so as to attack the parasites as they arrive at the bile ducts. Another reason for repeated treatment is, of course, the risk of new infection from pasture carrying cysts.

Within these limits, the effectiveness of the drug has been established by long experience and tested sometimes on a large scale. Parry (1959) treated 7400 sheep; the only side effects were lameness and accelerated heart beat for about half-an-hour following the injection.

Recovery of the growth rate of animals treated was established by Heida (1956). Only a little (up to 0·01 per cent) of the injected tetrachloride appears in the milk (especially the milk fat fraction); most of it within two days; all traces disappear after 10 days (Cieleszky and Kovacs, 1958).

Several Russian workers have published the results of extensive applications to large numbers of animals. Demidov (1957) treated 1018, Kagramanov (1955) 1728 and Zavgorodni (1955)

2512 infected sheep. In all cases excellent results, up to 100 per cent cures, were claimed. Side effects were few with 1–5 ml per animal. In one particular farm with over 5000 sheep, 135 were lost in 1957 due to fascioliasis. Carbon tetrachloride treatment

TABLE 13. COMPARATIVE RESULTS OF VARIOUS TREATMENTS TESTED BY MITTERPAK (1958) ON 9952 INFECTED SHEEP IN CZECHOSLOVAKIA

Preparation	Cures (%)	Average reduction in worm burden by (%)
Hexachlorethane (Motolit O)	73·7	61·8
Hexachlorethane (Igitol)	82·4	75·7
Carbon tetrachloride orally	90·5	68·4
Carbon tetrachloride subcut	6·1	52·2
Carbon tetrachloride and filicin (Distol express)	85·5	62·2
Carbon tetrachloride (Distol sheep)	59·9	45·9
Carbon tetrachloride 1 ml/25 kg subcut and 4 g hexachlorethane (Motolit O) orally	95·8	83·2

was given in November 1957, February 1958 and May 1958; there were no deaths in 1958. Pearson and Boray (1961) recommended at least 2 ml per 20 lb body weight for cattle (with a maximum of 30 ml). Another reporter (Dukchovshoi, 1956), stated that only 107 out of 13,000 sheep treated by injection showed side effects (shivering and "depression").

Yakouenko (1959) tested different doses of tetrachloride (dissolved in equal volume of vasdine). When lambs were injected with 2 ml and sheep with 3 ml, 16 per cent of the animals still had fluke eggs in the faeces and 21 per cent still had live parasites. Dose of 3 ml for lambs and 4–4·5 ml for sheep resulted in no eggs in faeces after the 9th day, and an absence of live worms. Rabbits were treated with 0·3 ml of CCl_4 per kg body weight (Ganasevitch and Skovronski, 1956); pigs of 15–84 kg weight were given 1–6 ml of 3:1 CCl_4 in liquid paraffin injected into the skin (Winterhalter and Delak, 1956 a, b and c) or 1 ml per 10 kg body weight (Kovacs and Nemeseri, 1957). Hyaluronidase injected intramuscularly increases the efficiency of carbon tetrachloride according to Winterhalter (1961). Carbon tetrachloride emulsion with local anaesthetic compounds has been produced in Germany as Ursodistol and was tested on large numbers of sheep with good results (Bühner and Pfeiffer, 1960; Bühner, 1961).

Harmful Effects of Carbon Tetrachloride

There are many reports of such effects. Dorsman (1959a) believed that to be effective, the drug has to be used at the rate of 15 mg/kg body weight (by mouth) which is a near-toxic amount for cattle. Winterhalter and Delak (1956 a and b) observed necrosis at the site of injection in cattle and hence considered the use of the drug in cattle impractical. Lameness may occur and last for a brief period (Parry, 1959; Yakovlev, 1955). Administering a full dose of 20 ml to several hundred cows, Veselova and Velikovskaya (1959) observed side effects in 20 per cent of the animals; these effects, appearing on the second day and lasting for 4–9 days, included a temperature rise of between 0·5 and 1·5°C, accelerated heart beat and breathing. An increase of leucocyte count and of urobilin level in the urine, occasionally even of bilirubin in the serum, were also detected. Komjäthy (1957) found the injection of pure tetrachloride preferable to the mixture with paraffin. No side effects were observed in buffaloes and equines in large scale trials in India; on the other hand there were toxic effects on fat tailed sheep (Sarwar and Barya, 1960).

One of the aftermaths of treatment is hypocalcaemia, and certain workers have recommended that for some weeks before treatment the animals be supplied with bone meal *ad lib*; or else with calcium preparations, or magnesium sulphate and linseed infusions (Slanina *et al.*, 1955; Kotlan and Kovacs, 1957).

Komjäthy (1957) and Kovacs (1959) advised a diet rich in carbohydrate before treatment; the latter author would exclude from treatment animals that are either very fat or undernourished.

Kovacs suggested adding to the mixture of liquid paraffin and carbon tetrachloride some Lidocaine base (diethyl amino 2–6 dimethyl acetanilid hydrochloride) at the rate of 0·5 g per cent — this helps to reduce the uneasiness of the animals after the treatment.

Despite the reports of side effects it would seem that improved techniques and precautions such as those cited above, can make the drug practically harmless to cattle. Taking the precautions quoted Kovacs (1958) was able to treat (by intramuscular injection on the side of the neck) no fewer than 150,000 cattle with only a small number showing any side effects. Repetition of treatment within 3–6 months was well tolerated. The rate of weight increase and milk yield picked up within days, and during the first few days, the milk contained no more than 3 mg of the drug per litre.

Similarly, Demidov and Veselova (1959) had only one fatality (an old and heavily infested animal) out of 10,000 cattle treated by subcutaneous injection. Recently, Kendall and Parfitt (1962) found that by increasing the dose above 2 ml per 100 lb of body weight they were able to kill relatively young flukes, i.e. those over 5–6 weeks old; but this result was not confirmed by Williams (1963).

On horses, carbon tetrachloride was used at the rate of 10–20 ml. in the adult and 6–10 ml in foals with good results (Ugron and Skovronski, 1959).

Mechanism of the Hepatotoxic Effects of Carbon Tetrachloride

The mechanism by which the drug damages the liver has recently been under investigation and discussion. Judah and Rees (1950) found that rat liver slices, tested 18 hr after poisoning with tetrachloride had lost, partly or wholly, the ability to oxidize a variety of substrates. The mitochondria in isolation showed the same property, and it was deduced that carbon tetrachloride damages the structure of liver mitochondria. The above changes can be detected as early as 5–10 hr after poisoning, and an accumulation of neutral fats in the liver can be detected within 3 hr. Sinha (cited by Judah and Rees) established the loss of soluble enzymes from the cells within 14–18 hr from administration of the drug.

Brody (1959) considered the changes in mitochondria as secondary to anoxia; this would be due to the drug (acting through the sympathetic nervous system) causing constriction of vessels to the liver. Furthermore, the drug would stimulate the production of epinephrine and norepinephrine which prolong the vaso-constriction. Adrenergic-blocking agents (ergotamine and phenoxybenzamine) counteract the effect of the drug on oxidations and on the accumulation of fat. Transection of the spinal cord (between the 2nd and 3rd thoracic vertebrae), reserpine and adrenalectomy, all have effects similar to these agents.

It has now been possible to separate two groups of effects of the carbon tetrachloride. If the anti-histaminic, phenergan, is injected intraperitoneally at the same time as the drug is given by stomach tube, some of the drug's effects are alleviated but others remain. Whilst fatty degeneration is not avoided, such symptoms as damage to mitochondria, leakage of calcium and enzymes, and necrosis are all greatly reduced. Again, adrenalectomy has the same effect (Rees *et al.,* 1961).

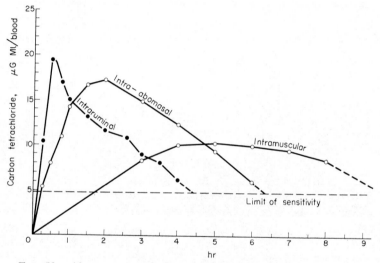

Fig. 59. Absorption of carbon tetrachloride into the blood, with different routes of administration in Merino ewes. (Condos, A. C. and McClymont, G. L., 1961).

A low level of the element selenium aggravates the effects of carbon tetrachloride. Two groups of 11 ewes each were fed a low selenium diet (oats and ladino clover), but one group was also given 0·1 ppm of sodium selenite. After 150 days on the experimental diets, all the animals were given 1 ml of carbon tetrachloride in a capsule. The group fed the selenite tolerated the dose well, but the other animals showed depression after 1–2 days, and one of them died. On autopsy, the peritoneal fluid was blood-stained, the liver parenchyma and gall bladder swollen and haemorrhagic. Selenium is in fact known to be involved in dietary hepatic necrosis; it acts in conjunction with vitamin E. In rats, vitamin E protects against the fatal deficiency of tocopherol caused by carbon tetrachloride (Hove, 1949; Schwarz, 1960).

The difference in toxicity of the carbon tetrachloride, depending on the route of administration, is now being systematically studied by Condos and McClymont (1961, 1963). The fall in plasma glutamic oxalacetic transaminase and isocitric dehydrogenase was used as one index of liver damage. This fall is about two times more severe after intraruminal as compared to intramuscular administration (Table 14). A fall of plasma calcium content is also noted, but corrects itself after about three days. The peak of drug level in the blood is reached within half an hour after intraruminal administration, within 2 hr after administration into the abomasum and within 4 hr after intramuscular injection (Fig. 59). Halogen from the drug could be detected in the expired air throughout the first 40–60 hours after treatment of the sheep used in these experiments (merino ewes). On the basis of the above enzymatic indices and also on other observations, the authors conclude that as little as 2 ml of carbon tetrachloride will cause some detectable damage to the liver, and that therefore the minimum effective dose should be used.

Hexachlorethane

Hexachlorethane is also widely used against fascioliasis, especially in cattle. Like carbon tetrachloride, it is ineffective against the migratory stages of the parasite, i.e. before the latter has reached the bile ducts. With regard to dosage, Potemkina (1945) found that 0·4 g per kg body weight cures up to 60 per cent of cases in cattle; higher doses are more effective, 0·8 g effecting complete cure. The milk remains tainted for 3 days after treatment.

The side effects of hexachlorethane include acute diffuse nephrosis, and slight degenerative changes in the liver parenchyma (Ehrlich et al., 1957; Ehrlich and Winterhalter, 1958); but all seem to be reversible within a week. According to Andraska (1959) they may be greatly reduced by preparing the animals on a

L

TABLE 14. MEAN VALUES OF GOT AND ICD ($\times 100$) ACTIVITIES IN THE PERIOD 20 TO 36 HOURS AFTER ADMINISTRATION OF CCl_4

Peak values are in italics.

(A. C. Condos and G. L. McClymont, 1963).

Route of administration and dose rate of CCl_4	GOT		
	Hours after administration of CCl_4		
	20	24	36
1. 2 ml IM	336 ± 44·9*	*447* ± 12·1	418 ± 9·5
2. 4 ml IM	481 ± 78·9	573 ± 68·2	*582* ± 64·6
3. 8 ml IM	915 ± 65·1	*986* ± 50·2	770 ± 60·2
4. 2 ml IR	645 ± 81·1	*801* ± 62·3	470 ± 64·2
5. 4 ml IR	990 ± 78·6	*1066* ± 53·5	668 ± 73·2
	ICD ($\times 100$)		
1. 2 ml IM	33 ± 8	*41* ± 2	22 ± 5
2. 4 ml IM	91 ± 33	*134* ± 24	34 ± 4
3. 8 ml IM	256 ± 30	*501* ± 22	268 ± 31
4. 2 ml IR	*342* ± 37·6	244 ± 36	51 ± 13
5. 4 ml IR	*594* ± 13	511 ± 31	254 ± 25

* Standard error.   IM, intramuscularly.   IR, intraruminally.

diet rich in calcium and vitamins but poor in fat and protein for 10 days before treatment.

Refuerzo (1947) used 10 g of hexachlorethane together with 1·75 g of Kamala extract per 30 kg of body weight for bovines, but to avoid side effects he split this amount into two doses given at least 2 days apart.

Other workers have used the drug in large doses, but administered it in a suspension with bentonite (Olsen, 1947, 1949; Schwartz, 1947). Adult cattle were drenched with 200 ml or more of this suspension, and the treatment was repeated twice a year. Occasionally an animal would show diarrhoea, dizziness and lack of appetite. The reason for this tolerance of high doses might lie in the fact that the drug is not readily soluble and hence is only slowly absorbed through the gut. Liver flukes implanted into rats under the skin are also killed by the drug reaching the skin through the circulation (Lienert, 1959 a and b).

In the case of horses, 0·2 g/kg had no effect; 0·4 g/kg disinfected the gastro-intestinal tract but increased the tonicity of the vagus nerve for 2–3 days; it also stimulated haemopoiesis and raised the chloride content of the blood. A dose of 7–10 mg/kg produced reversible toxic effects (Panasyuk, 1953). Diffuse nephrosis lasting about a week may be caused (Ehrlich and Winterhalter, 1958).

Side effects do not appear in sheep until dosage is raised to 20 mg/kg, while 40 mg/kg will cause the death of one in every 15 animals. A dose of 15–20 mg/kg is therefore recommended (Federmann, 1959). Lämmler (1956) found this compound preferable to carbon tetrachloride, filmaron oil, tartar emetic, emetine and antimony compounds (tests on rabbits).

Complete cure of pigs was effected with two doses of 0·2 g/kg with an interval of 2–4 weeks (Andreev, 1953). Hexachlorethane has also been used successfully on nutria (Polishchuk and Chuprinova, 1955).

There are favourable reports of the use of hexachlorethane in association with carbon tetrachloride, both given by mouth (Southcott, 1951; Grigoryan *et al.*, 1955; Khanbegyan, 1956). These tests have involved not only cattle but also sheep and goats, but the liver fluke carried by the animals was of the species *Fasciola gigantica*. It has been claimed that the mixture is effective against immature worms, too (Lungu *et al.*, 1959; 1960). It is interesting that hexachlorethane (at a high dose of 175 mg/kg) proved successful in a region of the Congo where carbon tetrachloride, atebrine and other drugs are reported to have been ineffective (Lederman, 1958). Veselova and Vorobev (1962) used 0·2 g/kg of hexachloroethane by mouth, and simultaneously gave 3·0–3·5 ml/100 kg of carbon tetrachloride in liquid paraffin (1:1) intramuscularly in cattle. They obtained 95–100 per cent cures, and also claimed that the mixture was effective against immature flukes. There were no side effects even with doses of 1 mg/kg and 8 ml/100 kg respectively.

Other Anthelminthics and Preparations

Ecobol, a preparation of carbon tetrachloride, was found

effective and harmless by Ullrich (1958; up to 300 mg/kg could be given to sheep) and Schmidt-Hoensdorf (1959). Other forms in which carbon tetrachloride is used include: *Carbaloma* — Sterile mixture of carbon tetrachloride, Diloma compound D and a local anaesthetic. At the rate of 18 ml this had no side effects on pregnant or recently calved cows (Jordan, 1960).

Difluorotetrachlorethane (also known as *Freon* or *Arcton*) was tested on 15 experimentally infected sheep of 60–70 kg at a dose of 20–30 ml given by intubation into the rumen. It was highly effective, but not active against immature worms (Demidov, 1955; Butyanov and Guzman, 1960). It can be mixed with some difluorodichlormethane to lower its melting point (Demidov, 1958). It can also be mixed with paraffin and administered by drench gun (Boray and Pearson, 1960). In tests on rats and rabbits this drug had no action against young flukes (Kendall and Parfitt, 1962) but eggs from treated cattle failed to develop beyond early cleavage, or did so only with great delay (Demidov, 1959).

Filixan (aqueous extract of male fern). Given by bottle to 8 experimentally infected sheep (dose 0·15–0·20 g/kg) this was 87·5 per cent effective (Demidov, 1955). Extensive tests of the efficacy of male fern extract were carried out by Norris (1925) and Montgomerie (1926).

Emetine Hydrochloride and Chlorquinine Diphosphate

These were given in combination by Basnuevo (1955) in human cases. A series of 10 daily injections of 0·025 g of the former and 0·25 g of the latter per ml of water were given intramuscularly. The adults were given 2–5 ml daily, and children 1 ml for every year of age with a maximum of 5 ml. Treatment is described as successful. The same author had earlier used the chlorquinine diphosphate in combination with quinacrine (Basnuevo 1954).

Hexachlorophene or G11 (2·2 methylene bis 3, 4, 6-trichlorophenol). This is injected subcutaneously or given orally, in olive oil. Based on an isolated observation by Hirschel, this treatment was tested on cattle by Dorsman (1959 a and b) and on sheep and cattle by Federmann (1959). Local inflammation persists for

2 weeks at the site of subcutaneous injection. A dose of 15 mg/kg body weight (or still better 20 mg) kills the flukes in the bile duct, but not the younger flukes in the liver. (However, 20 ml is the limit if harmful effects are to be avoided.) Pregnant ewes were also treated without bad effects (Boshan *et al.*, 1961).

At 40 mg/kg the compound acts against 5–9-week-old flukes in sheep and rabbits (Kendall and Parfitt, 1960).

Phenothiazine. This has been used as part of the preparation *Minel* which contains: 59·02 per cent phenothiazine, 39·34 per cent hexachloroethane, 82 per cent copper sulphate and 0·82 per cent cobalt sulphate. Güralp (1954) found it effective against a number of helminths, including *Fasciola hepatica* (and ineffective against many more). The dose used was 25 g for sheep, 18 g for lambs, 90 g for cattle, 25 g for goats, 15 g for kids.

Phenothiazine is not entirely free of toxic effects on farm animals, but sheep run a risk only if too young or undernourished. The drug appears to inhibit enzymes and in particular to cause uncoupling of oxidative phosphorylation in undernourished sheep; histologically, accumulation of fat in the liver cells is detected (Koch, 1963).

Bithionol (2,2′-dihydroxy-3,3′,5,5′-tetrachlorodiphenyl sulphide. Orally (75 mg/kg) 100 per cent successful in tests on sheep, but again not active against younger flukes even at 200 mg/kg (Ueno *et al.*, 1959).

Hetol (1,4 bis-trichlormethyl benzol) used at 150 mg/kg (or more), in sheep and 136 mg/kg in cattle, given by mouth in suspension in water. Well tolerated, provided animals are kept off fresh beet and cabbage 1 day before and 3 days after treatment (Behrens, 1960; Enigk and Düwel, 1960; Lämmler, 1960). The last author recommended a mixture of this preparation with phenothiazine (Lämmler, 1961).

Atebrin. In water or 25 per cent glucose given intravenously or intraperitoneally (one or two doses, 5–25 mg/kg). Causes transitory vagotony. Ehrlich *et al.* (1960b) made the important claim that this compound attacks the young flukes in the liver parenchyma. In tests *in vitro* Kurelěc *et al.* (1961) found that atebrin enters the parasite by both the mouth and the body surface, and spreads into various tissues of the worm (Fig. 60).

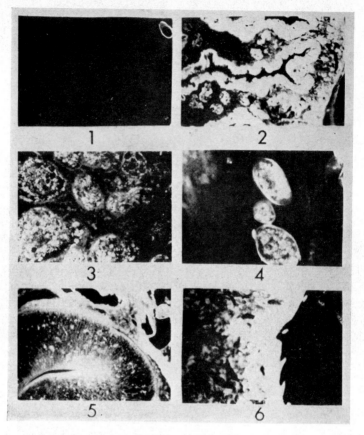

Fig. 60. Sections of adult liver flukes, after treatment *in vitro* with atebrin, showing the fluorescence of this drug under ultraviolet light (Kurelec *et al.,* 1961).

(1) control untreated. The other sections show the unequal distribution of atebrin, high in the: gut and yolk glands (2), testes (3), egg shells (4), sucker musculature (5) and tegument and muscle layers (6).

4,4-*diamino diphenyl methane*. In the form of hydrochloride administered orally to rabbits, this compound proved effective against immature flukes as well as adults, but unfortunately it is toxic to cattle (Williams, 1963).

CHAPTER 16

IMMUNOLOGICAL RESPONSE OF
THE HOST

MANY attempts have been made to produce antisera that on injection to farm animals, would either impart immunity to liver fluke infection (passive immunization), or else induce the formation of protective antibodies in the animals themselves (active immunization).

Demonstration of Antibodies

Perhaps the first relevant investigation on record is that of Guerrini (1908). He showed that the serum of a goat carrying liver flukes formed a precipitate when mixed with an aqueous extract of the parasite. This experiment corresponds to a rough precipitin test, demonstrating that the infected goat had formed antibodies to some components of the liver fluke tissue.

In order to induce the possible production of antibodies, an extract of the parasite's tissues is injected into a healthy animal. If the extract contains antigenic components, antibodies may become detectable in the serum. Kerr and Petkovitch (1935) used a 1 per cent suspension of dried powdered liver fluke tissue for injection into rabbits. (The eggs were teased out of the flukes and were not included.) The extract was injected into 7 rabbits, in nine doses of 1 ml every second day. Sera were obtained 1, 2 and 3 weeks after the end of the injections and were tested with the extract. They all gave positive precipitin reactions. It was concluded that the animals had formed antibodies to the liver fluke.

Ineffectiveness of Antibodies

In the experiments of Kerr and Petkovitch, the 7 immunized and another 3 control rabbits were infected with 13 metacercaria each, about a month after the end of the injections. The results of autopsies are given in Table 15. It appears that the immunized rabbits were indeed resistant to the infection to some extent. Furthermore, they contained no eggs in the faeces, whilst the unimmunized group not only harboured more worms but also released eggs of the parasite. One of the flukes in rabbit 2, and both in rabbit 3 were found to be "calcified".

TABLE 15.   EFFECT OF IMMUNIZATION BY THE INJECTION OF LIVER FLUKE ANTIGENS INTO RABBITS SUBSEQUENTLY INFECTED WITH 13 METACERCARIA EACH (KERR AND PETKOVITCH, 1935)

Rabbit number and treatment	Days after last injection at *post mortem*	Number of liver flukes recovered
(a) Immunized rabbits		
No. 1	92	1
2	92	1
3	92	2
4	92	2
5	103	2
6	103	2
7	118	3
(b) Non-immunized rabbits		
8	111	5
9	116	9
10	124	11

The results of Shibanai *et al.* (1956) point in the same direction. These workers prepared a vaccine from liver flukes and injected it into rabbits by various routes. About 70 days later the rabbits were infected; after another 56 days, autopsies showed that the damage caused to the liver by the liver flukes was less severe than in unimmunized controls. All the same, the development of the parasite was not affected by the vaccination.

In contrast to the above, most other workers have obtained negative results in their efforts to produce active immunization. However, in all cases antibodies were produced and could be detected by the precipitin or other tests.

Urquhart, Mulligan and Jennings (1954) prepared an antigen

in the way described in Appendix II and gave a series of injections to rabbits. In the end the rabbit sera contained antibodies giving the precipitin reaction. The precipitate was found to contain 0·155–1·17 mg/ml of nitrogen. This rose to 0·5–1·9 mg, after infection of the same animals with 50 cercarial cysts, as compared with 0·2 mg in controls (infected but not immunized). However, these precipitins did not hinder the establishment of the parasite in the host.

Similar results were obtained by Healey (1955a). Rabbits immunized with fluke extract were infected, and killed 35 days later. There was no difference in the number of parasites in the experimental and the control groups. Nevertheless, some antibody was again present as shown by a skin test which was positive in all immunized rabbits. The positive reaction could be elicited with antigen from *Fasciola hepatica,* and from *F. magna,* but not with antigen from *Schistosoma mansoni.*

At the 16th International Veterinary Congress, Ershov (1959) described work carried out at the Moscow Institute of Helminthology, which is of particular interest as: (a) it was carried out on a large scale, (b) the animals used were sheep and not rabbits, (c) it was carried out concurrently with work against other parasites, and (d) the active components of the antigens were isolated. The method used for the preparation of antigens from the liver fluke is set out in Appendix II.

Antigens were injected subcutaneously or intramuscularly into 97 lambs, which were subsequently given cysts of the parasite at intervals. Only 10–25 per cent of the animals resisted the infection, and these only for up to 45 days after the end of the injections. Some others showed partial resistance.

Attenuated Larvae as Antigen Carriers

Immunization of animals against parasites may also be elicited in certain cases by exposure to live parasites that have been so treated as to become unable to establish themselves in the host; in this way, immunization may be achieved without all the damage of actual infestation, and also without the necessity of isolating antigens for injection. Jarrett and co-workers (1958) achieved great success with this method against the parasite,

Dictyocaulus viviparus, which causes parasitic bronchitis in cattle. Larvae of the parasite were irradiated with doses of X-rays that left them alive and capable of infiltrating the host but incapable of developing further in it. Larvae so "attenuated" were then used for "infecting" healthy animals, so as to elicit the immune reaction in them and thus protect them against later raw infection. The same research workers also studied *Fasciola hepatica* and *Fasciola gigantica*, but no results concerning these parasites were published.

Later, other workers approached the task. Hughes (1962; 1963) irradiated cysts with doses which caused the metacercaria to remain stunted and to become encysted readily in the host liver. Two thousand to four thousand r attenuate the cysts to the extent that mice infected with them survive. The larvae do reach the liver but die 18–28 days later, having reached a size of only 1 mm, as against the normal 4–5 mm. However, infection with these attenuated larvae did not result in reduced infectivity on subsequent challenge with normal cysts.

The same form of attenuation was used by Wikerhauser (1961). The doses used were much larger; 5000 to 20,000 r made the cysts unable to develop in the rabbit, whilst lower doses (3000–8000 r) permitted development. Intermediate doses (about 12,000 r) permitted the cysts to produce mature flukes but the eggs from these failed to produce miracidia.

Thorpe and Broome (1962) administered a dose of 40 irradiated cysts to rats and at autopsy ten days later recovered: 6·8 flukes for a dose of 1000 r, 0·4 flukes for a dose of 2500 r, and none for higher doses. Animals given these attenuated larvae were challenged some weeks later with 20 unirradiated metacercaria each. The results of autopsy after another 10 weeks were as follows:

Dose in r given to attenuated cysts	1000	2500	5000	7500	10,000
Number of flukes recovered 17 weeks later	7·7	2·7	4·3	4·5	6·7

Although the reason for the phenomenon is not clear, it is interesting that more satisfactory results could be obtained by delaying the challenge for another two weeks, when the number of flukes recovered were respectively 6·6, 1·1, 0·3, 0·4 and 1·5 for the same attenuating doses as above.

It would appear from these results that the entry of attenuated metacercaria imparts a certain degree of immunity, provided the radiation dose used for the attenuation is neither too low nor too high.

Conclusion

The experiments reviewed in this chapter have established the fact that the mammalian host does produce antibodies to liver fluke antigens, whether these are injected after separation *in vitro* or are carried by the live parasite. These antibodies are detectable by precipitin and other tests, but they fail to impart any real protection to the mammal against subsequent infection.

CHAPTER 17

DIAGNOSTIC TESTS*

FROM the investigations discussed in the previous chapter it may be concluded that antibodies to the liver fluke are undoubtedly produced, but that for some reason they are not capable of stemming the infection, and cannot as yet be put to therapeutic use.

However, since these antibodies are easily detectable, their presence may at least be used for the diagnosis of fascioliasis in cases where the infection is suspected, but cannot be confirmed by the detection of eggs in the faeces.

Several such diagnostic tests have been developed. Some are based on the precipitin reaction, but others are based on allergic reactions to liver-fluke extracts. Although the exact extent to which allergic reactions are due to typical antibodies is an unsolved problem, the tests involved are described as immunological and are discussed below with the precipitin reactions.

Precipitin Reaction

This is based of course on the property of antibodies to form a precipitate if mixed with soluble antigen. The precipitate contains both antigen and antibody, but in most cases it consists mainly of antibody. Often the antiserum is left undiluted and is tested against successive dilutions of the antigen; the largest dilution that will still give a visible precipitate is described as the titer of the serum.

In the tests under discussion, sera from infected animals are tested with liver fluke antigen and compared with sera from unifected animals. A group of Japanese workers (Ichihara *et al.,* 1956 a, b and c) who recently investigated the precipitin reaction

* See also Chapter 18.

in some detail, concluded that (in both cattle and goats) a positive precipitin reaction indicates the existence of liver fluke infection with an accuracy of 90 per cent. The amount of precipitate however cannot serve as an indication of the severity of the infection, i.e. of the number of the parasites.

Flocculation Test

Sterols are added to the antigen in some immunological tests, such as the Wasserman test, in order to "sensitize" the antigen. The sterols are serologically unreactive and an explanation of their effect is that they become coated with antigen; thus they form large particles with the antigen-antibody molecules, making the precipitate or flocculate more obvious. Suessenguth and Kline (1944) have used crystals of cholesterol for the flocculation test for trichinosis. This type of test has been adjusted to the liver fluke work, mainly by Japanese workers. Komine et al. (1955) found that the positive reaction is more pronounced in the case of older infected animals, perhaps (they suggest) on account of the larger amounts of serum protein in the blood. Susumi et al. (1958; 1959) have tested a variety of modifications and concluded that the minimum titer detectable by this test is 1:32.

The procedure for this test is as follows: 1 per cent cholesterol solution in absolute alcohol is added to a small amount of water, and shaken. The antigen is also added and shaken; this is followed by addition of a NaCl solution. The resulting emulsion contains crystals coated with the antigen. The serum to be tested is heated at 56°C for 30 min, and then pipetted into the antigen mixture. The whole test can be carried out with very small amounts, so that 0·05 ml of serum is adequate; it is placed (with a pipette) in the chamber of a paraffin-ringed slide, and a drop of the antigen emulsion is added. The slide is rotated flat for a few minutes and is then examined under the microscope at a magnification of × 100, with the light cut down. Where the reaction is positive the crystals become clumped together, where it is negative they remain dispersed. It is helpful to dye the crystals with azur III, malachite green or light green.

Micro-precipitin Test

A test described as micro-precipitin was developed by Wiker-hauser and co-workers. Excysted live metacercaria are immersed in the sera to be tested for antibodies. If such antibodies are in fact present a "precipitate" forms around the cercaria, and especially around the mouth and excretory pore. In tests with sera from 163 cattle, 95·6 per cent of those with fascioliasis produced these precipitates; but sera from 18 per cent of uninfected animals did the same (Wikerhauser et al., 1961; Wikerhauser, 1961).

Complement Fixation Test

Generally, when antigen combines with antibody, another factor in the serum, called complement, also enters the complex.

All three — antigen, antibody and complement — combine physically and a point will come when all the available complement will have been removed from the serum into the precipitate.

In the complement fixation test the question asked is whether the serum tested contains or not antibodies to particular antigen say for example to liver fluke antigen. If the antigen is added in a tube to the serum under test, the complement will be removed from this serum if there is antibody, and will not be removed if no complex is formed. The removal or fixation of the complement cannot however be directly seen, so that some means of detecting its removal or its continued presence is now required.

This means is provided by sensitized foreign red cells. These are red cells which have been pre-treated with red cell haemolysins. This pre-treatment or sensitization leaves the red cells still intact, but renders them liable to immediate lysis if they are transferred into a serum containing complement. In other words, haemolysins alone react with red cells in some way but do not break them, but when complement is also added the lysis occurs. If now such sensitized red cells are added to the test tube where the serum and the liver-fluke antigen were mixed, they will be lysed if complement is still available; this will mean that no antigen-antibody reaction had occurred, or that the serum contained no antibody to that antigen. If the cells are not lysed, the complement must have been removed and for that to happen antibody must have been present.

The controls will consist of tubes with serum alone, and others with the antigen alone, to which red cells are added. Of course, removal of all the complement will depend on the presence of sufficient antigen, and the optimal dilutions of antigen will have to be determined by titration.

This kind of test has been carried out by many investigators attempting to establish that a positive reaction is indeed specific to liver fluke infection, in which case the test could be used diagnostically (Paccanaro, 1909, on sheep; Weinberg, 1909, on sheep; Servantie, 1921, on sheep; Höppli, 1921, on sheep and bovines; Brocq-Rousseau, Cauchemez and Urbain, 1923, on sheep; Wagner, 1935, on sheep). To these should be added some tests on human patients (Bacigalupo, 1934). The results of this earlier work are not all in agreement, but the procedures for obtaining antigens were varied, some experiments included no controls, and furthermore sheep that gave a positive reaction but carried no liver fluke may have carried the parasite at some earlier stage.

Using a saline extract, Bénex *et al.* (1959) found that whilst a negative complement fixation test reliably excludes fascioliasis, a positive reaction does not necessarily mean that this parasite is present; the positive reaction with liver fluke antigen can also be obtained where not *Fasciola* but another fluke, *Dicrocoelium dendriticum*, is present.

Diagnostic Tests Based on Hypersensitivity — Skin Tests

Host reactions to a particular parasite find their expression not only in the formation of typical antibodies such as precipitins, but also in the development of a state of hypersensitivity. If the host is challenged with extracts of the parasite, it reacts to them abnormally, whilst the same extracts are harmless to and elicit no reaction from uninfected individuals. Such reactions, if immediate, are called anaphylactic, allergic, hypersensitivity or atopic reactions. Obviously, allergic reactions are evidence of the (current or recent) existence of the parasite within the host, and provide a possible basis for diagnostic tests.

Typically, the reactions are elicited by applying the antigen or injecting it into the skin, when redness, weals, indurations and other local changes become obvious within a brief period of time.

Soulsby (1954) was able to transfer the hypersensitive state to uninfected animals by injecting serum from the infected individuals. He also found that he could desensitize a small area of the skin by repeated small injections, but could not achieve general desensitization.

In their efforts to establish whether the allergic reactions occur as a response to liver-fluke antigens and if so, whether they are specific, the early workers harvested conflicting results. Sievers and Oyarzoun (1932) obtained encouraging results from an experiment with 100 sheep, on which they applied skin and intradermal tests one day before slaughter.

For the skin test, they scarified both thighs and rubbed one with antigen (in a paste with glycerine), the other with glycerine alone. The antigens used were of three kinds; sixty sheep were rubbed with dried powdered liver flukes, twenty with an ether-extract of this powder, and another twenty with a chloroform-extract of the same.

For the intradermal test, they used a saline extract (prepared as specified in Appendix II) for all 100 animals.

At autopsy, all animals that had given positive reactions were found to carry the parasite; all animals proved free of the parasite had given negative reactions. Since all three extracts were equally effective, the antigens involved in the skin reaction must be soluble in ether and chloroform. The actual numbers were as follows:

Animals giving a positive reaction:

Skin test with powder-antigen	33
Skin test with ether-extract	16
Skin test with chloroform extract	12
Intradermal test	20

On the other hand, Wagner (1935) failed to obtain an anaphylactic reaction from some sheep that definitely released parasite eggs in the faeces. Conversely, Curasson (1931) recorded positive reactions from 10 that were free of the parasite.

Soulsby (1954) skin-tested 212 cattle with liver-fluke antigen prepared by the method of Trawinski (Appendix II). 164 cattle formed a weal 5–6 mm wide with thickening of the skin; all these proved on autopsy a day later to be infected. Seven cattle that only formed a weal without thickening of the skin and 41 that gave no reaction whatsoever, all proved to be free of parasites.

Another test on 219 cattle was carried out in Puerto Rico (Rivera-Anaya *et al.*, 1953). Out of 195 animals with liver fluke eggs in the faeces, 56 per cent gave positive precipitin and 95 per cent positive intradermal reactions. The latter were described as positive where a weal of at least 18×15 mm appeared within half-an-hour of the injection.

A test with *F. gigantica* antigen on 40 cattle also showed perfect correlation of presence of infection and positive reaction (Patnaik and Das, 1961). Four animals with no fluke but with scarred liver also gave a positive reaction, a result easily explicable on past infection.

The antigen can be diluted greatly, up to 1:100,000 (Minning and Vogel, 1950) and in fact an antigen that is diluted only (for example) 1:1000 or less is far too strong (Sobiegh, 1951).

Mihaescu *et al.* (1953) also confirms the usefulness of the intradermal tests in cattle. In their tests, two-thirds of infected bovines gave a positive reaction; also about half of those that carried no liver flukes at the time but had lesions betraying previous infections (angiocholitis, cirrhosis). It is interesting that some animals with hepatic degeneration and congestion (lesions not associated with liver fluke disease) also gave a positive reaction. In these tests the antigen was an extract from whole flukes obtained by treatment with NaOH.

As a variant of the skin test, some workers used the palpebral test, injecting the antigen into the eyelid. Positive cases react within 15–45 min with a soft painful flat oedema, red at the centre. This soon retreats but becomes replaced by a larger oedema reaching its maximum at 4 hr and persisting for 7–8 hr. Szaflarski (1950, 1951) and Sobiegh (1951) obtained good diagnostic results from this test using the polysaccharide fraction of the antigen; the protein fraction proved unsuitable. In some experiments this form of the test proved unreliable in that it disagreed with the results of the intradermal test (Fedyushin and Ytechev 1952).

Gonzales *et al.* (1950) injected the antigen in the vaginal and caudal folds of 30 cows known to shed liver fluke eggs, and in a group of controls. All animals developed an indurated weal. In infected animals this was $1 \cdot 5$–3 cm^2 in size, but was smaller and

M

less indurated in the control group. Furthermore, the infected group had a red papule in the middle of the induration. Fasciola antigens are now commercially available; those prepared by freeze-drying of the tissue may be quicker-acting than those prepared by heat drying (Ono *et al.*, 1956).

A Comparison of Tests

The two main diagnostic tests were compared on a large scale by Babenskas *et al.* (1958) in Lithuania. This group of investigators was able to work on 2996 cattle that were definitely infected with the liver fluke. The percentage detection was as follows:

Agglutination test	87·5%
Intradermal test	74·5%
Detection of eggs in faeces	37·5%

In Kellaway's (1928) experiments, a saline extract was responsible for the allergic reactions, and an alcoholic extract for the complement fixation.

The Rabbit as Antiserum Producer

It has been established by Trawinski (1959) that antibodies to the liver fluke produced by the rabbit in response to fluke antigens are in fact suitable for the precipitin, complement fixation and intradermal diagnostic reactions and tests on other species. He carried out his tests on 170 cows and 340 sheep, of which 108 and 296 respectively were definitely parasitized by the liver fluke, as confirmed at slaughter. The results of the tests were 85 per cent or more accurate.

Cross Reactions

Several authors have claimed that animals with fascioliasis may give a positive reaction to the tuberculin test, an eventuality that reduces the value of the diagnostic test for tuberculosis (Merlen, 1950; Kochnev, 1950 on cattle with liver flukes localized in the lungs; Fedyushin and Ytechev, 1952). Again, others have failed to confirm the cross reaction (Manukyan, 1955; Kokurichev and Karbainov, 1957). However, the experiments described by Fedyushin and Ytechev are thorough, and they showed that the cross reaction could be abolished (at least in a number of cases) by treating the animals with anthelminthics for fascioliasis (Tables 16 and 17).

Kokurichev and Karbainov did in fact obtain a positive or doubtful reaction to tuberculin from some animals not suffering from tuberculosis; but of these some did and others did not

TABLE 16. POSITIVE REACTION TO TUBERCULIN OF CATTLE FREE OF TUBERCULOSIS BUT CARRYING THE LIVER FLUKE. DOUBLE-INJECTION TUBERCULIN TEST (FEDYUSHIN AND YTECHEV, 1952)

Age of animals	Number	First injection						Second injection					
		+		±		−		+		±		−	
		ID	P	ID	P	ID	P	ID	P	ID	P	ID	P
Adult	832	20	—	56	5	756	825	83	15	114	34	638	783
Calves	58	—		—		58		—		—		58	

ID = intradermal test; P = palpebral test. No palpebral test was carried out on the 58 calves.

TABLE 17. RESULTS OF TUBERCULIN TEST REPEATED AFTER THE CATTLE WERE TREATED WITH TWO INJECTIONS OF HEXACHLOROETHANE WITH AN INTERVAL OF 3 MONTHS (FEDYUSHIN AND YTECHEV, 1952)

Reaction to tuberculin before treatment	Numbers	Reaction to tuberculin after treatment and reaction of untreated controls					
		+		±		−	
		ID	P	ID	P	ID	P
(a) Treated animals:							
Positive	28	2	—	9	3	17	25
Doubtful	13	1	—	6	—	6	13
(b) Untreated controls:							
Positive	2	1	—	1	—	—	2
Calves, negative	3	—	—	—	—	—	3

ID = intradermal test; P = palpebral test.

carry the liver fluke, so that the hypersensitivity to tuberculin might be attributable to some other unknown cause.

The reverse cross reaction has also been recorded by Soulsby (1954); animals suffering from tuberculosis reacted positively to liver fluke antigen.

Cattle harbouring several other parasites give no cross reaction with liver fluke antigens; Sobiegh (1951) carried out skin tests on 168 cattle and listed the following parasites as showing no cross reaction: *Dicrocoelium dendriticum, Moniezia, Trichostrongylus, Nematodirus* and *Trichuris*. Mihaescu *et al.* (1953) confirmed this in the case of *Dicrocoelium*. However, Benex *et al.* obtained cross reactions in complement fixation tests with sera from sheep infected with either *Fasciola hepatica* or *Dicrocoelium*.

A positive skin reaction is also given by cattle carrying the liver fluke if challenged with antigens from *Schistosoma* (Minning and Vogel, 1950).

Fractionation of Antigens

For the purpose of discovering the immunologically active components of liver fluke extracts, several groups of workers undertook their fractionation. The fractions were assessed for activity in precipitin tests by some workers and in complement fixation or intradermal tests by others.

Minning and Fuhrmann (1955) split the extract into protein, carbohydrate and lipoid fractions, the last sub-divided into total, ether-soluble, acetone-soluble and chloroform-soluble lipids. In complement fixation tests the carbohydrate fraction was inactive and the lipid fractions were very weak; the protein fraction was active but not as much as the whole alcoholic extract of liver-fluke tissue. This was further confirmed by Gomes and Lavier (1956). Even the dried-up contents of saline where liver flukes had been kept for one day previously were active as antigens if re-dissolved in water (Minning *et al.*, 1958).

Ichihara *et al.* (1956a and b) split the liver fluke extract into five fractions: polysaccharide, methanol-soluble lipids, methanol-soluble lipids after removal of a precipitate appearing when the fraction is kept for two days in the refrigerator, ethanol-soluble lipids, and ethanol-soluble lipids after removal of the precipitate forming after two days in the refrigerator. Each one of these fractions gives no reaction (or a very weak one) in precipitin tests with sera from infected animals; but a combination of the poly-saccharide and lipid fractions gives abundant precipitate.

Active principles for intradermal tests were separated by Ono and Watanabe (1956) and by Maekawa *et al.* (1954) (Appendix II). The material obtained by the first group was described as "glycogen fraction" but was shown to be a polysaccharide other than glycogen, protein-free and producing fructose and glucose on hydrolysis. The second group obtained a "crystalline fraction V", soluble in phenol, acetic acid and ammonia, but only slightly soluble in water or organic solvents. This fraction elicits an intradermal reaction within 15–30 min of injection. It contains protein, and was shown to be rich in aspartic acid and valine but to lack methionine, phenylalanine, isoleucine and proline (Table 18).

TABLE 18. AMINOACID COMPOSITION OF THE COMPONENT OF LIVER FLUKE EXTRACT ELICITING ALLERGIC DERMO-REACTION (MAEKAWA AND KUSHIBE, 1955)

Aminoacid	Amount in g per 100 g of the antigen	Relative per molecule
Glycine	5·830	21
Alanine	7·073	21
Valine	6·689	18
Leucine	14·220	29
Cystine	2·618	3
Arginine	6·991	11
Histidine	4·796	9
Lysine	2·618	5
Aspartic acid	8·241	17
Glutamic acid	12·431	23
Serine	5·294	14
Threonine	6·144	14
Oxyproline	0·490	1
Tyrosine	5·434	8
Tryptophane	2·200	3

The results tend to show that different fractions may be differentially active in various tests, and that both protein and carbohydrate may be capable of eliciting the allergic response.

It might also be expected that reactions to liver fluke extract will vary with the time that has elapsed from the initiation of infection. Biguet, Capron and Tran Van Ky (1962) were able to demonstrate 15 antigenic components in liver fluke extract by agar gel immunoelectrophoresis. The antibodies appeared in the serum of rabbits, given injections of crude liver fluke extract, in a specific sequence shown in Fig. 61.

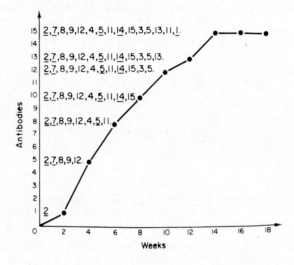

FIG. 61. Order of appearance in the rabbit serum of the fractions of antibody to the liver fluke (Biguet, Capron and Tran Van Ky, 1962). The numbers refer to the fractions 1–15 separated by agar gel immuno-electrophoresis. Those underlined are specific to the liver fluke.

CHAPTER 18

HUMAN FASCIOLIASIS

SEVERAL hundred cases of human fascioliasis from all parts of the world have been described in medical journals. The largest single outbreak on record is perhaps that in the Lyons area of France in 1956–57. The majority of cattle in the area were infested in that year, and concurrently about 500 human cases were diagnosed (Wibaut-Isebree Moens, 1958).

The symptoms appearing in human fascioliasis include digestive upsets, pain, fever, leucocytosis with a most characteristic strong eosinophilia, and an excess of γ-globulin in the plasma (Deschiens and Bénex, 1960). Urticaria and anaemia (Facey and Marsden, 1960), and loss of weight and sweating (Dysou, 1959), were noted. Hepatomegaly sets in at a late stage (Claisse and Hartmann, 1954). Gallstones are described as a frequent complication (Faiguenbaum et al., 1958; Derom et al., 1956). Calcifications in the gall bladder and obstructive jaundice may complicate surgery (Faiguenbaum et al., 1958), hence treatment with anthelminthics such as emetine hydrochloride is preferable, and effective.

As in other animals, the parasite may occasionally be found in unusual locations: in subcutaneous nodules in the abdominal wall (Hevia et al., 1958) and even in the brain (Lunedei et al., 1934); or in the lungs or bronchi as in a case from Hawaii where a patient coughed up a worm (Alicata, 1953b). In Syria where raw liver is sometimes consumed, the worm may become attached to the pharynx (Watson and Kerim, 1956). Callot and Gayot (1946) pointed out that the flukes do not survive if left in the liver after slaughter of the host for more than seven hours.

Cases on record from Britain were reviewed by Facey and Marsden (1960), who also gave a complete account of an outbreak of six cases in Ringwood, Hampshire, in the autumn of 1958. In this part of the Avon valley almost all cattle in some herds are infected and the prevalence of the parasite precludes the rearing of sheep. There are in addition natural beds of watercress, and it is to the eating of this cress in the wet summer of 1958 that all six cases can be attributed. The authors gave the case histories and also set out the results of laboratory tests (Table 19).

The acute phase of the disease is characterized by allergic, immunological and toxic reactions, typically taking the following course: after a transitory period of dyspepsia with or without slight fever, more severe symptoms set in abruptly; the temperature oscillates and may reach 40°C, and there is very strong abdominal pain. Fever, associated with enlargement of the liver, and excessive eosinophilia, are proposed as a triad of symptoms of diagnostic value. Urticaria episodes may occur, the skin acquiring an "earthy" colour resembling that in Addison's disease. Splenomegaly may develop, probably in association with ectopic localization of parasites; if this involves the lungs there will be a cough and other respiratory symptoms.

Asthenia, wasting and digestive upsets are frequent sequels. The flukes may become calcified in the liver, the calcification being detectable by radiography; or, they may pass to the bile ducts, in which case the latent phase of the disease sets in.

In this phase the symptoms are few, but the obstruction, irritation and pathological thickening of the bile ducts (described by Biggart, 1937) may (depending on the number of flukes present) lead to biliary cirrhosis and to secondary bacterial infections. Relapses of the acute phase may occur, presumably due to flukes re-entering the liver tissue.

Facey and Marsden treated their patients with chloroquine sulphate or hydroxychloroquine sulphate. The drugs were badly tolerated, and, although the acute symptoms subsided, the flukes were not killed; 5 of the 6 patients continued to pass fluke eggs in the faeces (detected by the method of Ridley and Hawgood, 1956, see p. 199). Emetine was used in case 3 following a relapse, and after this treatment the ova disappeared from the faeces.

Diagnostic Tests

The applicability of immunological diagnostic tests (such as those discussed in the preceding chapter) to human fascioliasis has long interested investigators on the Continent.

TABLE 19. HUMAN FASCIOLIASIS: RESULTS OF BLOOD AND OTHER TESTS ON SIX HUMAN CASES IN AN OUTBREAK AT RINGWOOD, HAMPSHIRE, AUTUMN 1958 (FACEY AND MARSDEN, 1960)

	Case 1				Case 2			Case 3		Case 4		Case 5		Case 6	
Date of onset of symptoms:	20/12/58				17/12/58			3/11/58		1/8/58		8/12/58		30/1/59	
	Oct 58	Dec 58	Jan 59	Mar 59	Jan 59	Feb 59	May 59	Feb 59	Apr 59	Mar 59	May 59	June 59	Sept 59	Apr 59	July 59
Haemoglobin (%)	104	100	80	78	94	108	88	87	—	75	83	95	86	75	88
Haemoglobin (g/100 ml)	15·2	14·6	11·7	11·4	13·7	15·8	12·8	12·7	—	11·0	12·1	13·9	12·5	11·0	12·9
Leucocytes (c, mm)	5900	4600	—	5200	7400	9000	6100	9100	—	9500	6500	7000	3710	14000	6700
Eosinophils (%)	2	19	29	45	47	32	28	24	—	44	9	32	9	8	11
Eosinophils (c, mm)	118	874	—	2340	3478	2880	1708	2184	—	4180	585	2240	333	4000	737
E.S.R. Wintrobe (mm/hr)	3	29	47	49	15	21	43	15	—	38	14	46	16	43	10
Thymol units	—	—	6	5	—	—	1	4	—	—	—	—	—	—	1
Alk. phosphatase units	—	—	18	19	—	—	31	9	—	—	—	—	—	—	6
Bilirubin (mg/100 ml)	—	1·0	0·8	0·5	—	—	1·2	0·5	—	—	—	—	—	—	0·8
C.F.T.	—	—	—	+++	Neg.	+++	+	+++	+	+++	+	++	+	Neg.	+++
Fasciola hepatica eggs in faeces	—	—	Neg.	+ (Feb 6)		+		+		+++					Neg.

The earliest tests of Bacigalupo (1934) and Rukawina (1935) were inconclusive. About a decade later, Lavier and Stefanopoulo (1944) prepared antigens by the procedure described in Appendix II, and carried out complement fixation and intradermal tests on 5 patients with fascioliasis; other patients, not harbouring the parasite, provided controls.

In the complement fixation test, only the fascioliasis patients gave a positive reaction (including one patient who had been cured five months earlier). These results indicate that antibodies to the liver fluke are produced by man, a conclusion in agreement with that from animal experimentation. Similarly, Minning and Vogel (1950) obtained a positive reaction from three children carrying the parasite, even six months after cure. However, antigens from digestive glands of infected snails and from cercaria of *Bilharzia* also gave positive reactions (although adult *Bilharzia* gave negative reactions).

In the allergic tests Lavier and Stefanopoulo observed (within a few minutes of intradermal injection) a weal 1–3 cm wide and surrounded by an erythema in 5 or the persons tested. This disappeared within 1–2 hr, but an infiltration of the skin persisted for a further 4–6 hr. The whole reaction is obliterated within the day, but some urticaria or pain at the nearest joint may persist. Actually some of Lavier's positive patients reacted much more violently to the injection; one developed cardio-vascular shock, nausea and diarrhoea; another became pale for 15 min. The results were satisfactory because the 5 positive patients were known to harbour the liver fluke, and all 6 controls gave a negative reaction. Amongst the latter was a syphilitic; a cross reaction of syphilitic serum and liver-fluke antigen at particular concentrations, resulting in a pseudo-positive reaction, has been claimed by Servantie (1921), Höppli (1922) and Bettancourt and Borges (1922).

Further tests were undertaken by Morenas (1944); Mazotti (1948); Monnet *et al.* (1950, 1951), and Coudert (1952). All concluded that the intradermal test is a sensitive and specific method of diagnosis, particularly useful where no eggs are found in the faeces, but where fascioliasis is suspected on the grounds that bacterial infections have been excluded and yet a marked and progressive eosinophilia persists. The absence of eggs from the faeces may be due to the presence of the immature (migratory stage) of the parasite, or to its calcification in the liver or ectopic localization in other tissues.

An intradermal reaction can also be obtained with metabolic products released by the worm in saline *in vitro* (Wikerhauser and Bartulic, 1961).

Biagi *et al.* (1958) applied the intradermal and precipitin tests to 468 persons chosen at random. Whilst 27·7 per cent gave a positive intradermal, only 4 per cent showed a positive precipitin reaction. These persons were from an area of Mexico where fascioliasis is endemic. In contrast, the proportion of positive reactions among students in Mexico City was 14·3 per cent and 1·4 per cent. Only 5 out of 252 persons who had a positive skin test had eggs in the faeces. Of 7 established cases of fascioliasis, 6 had a positive precipitin reaction and all 7 had positive skin reactions.

It is the conclusion of these authors that skin tests may be useful in epidemiological surveys for identifying suspected cases, but that only a positive precipitin reaction at an antigen dilution of 1:5000 or over can establish a case with certainty.

Immunoelectrophoresis

An attempt to detect the presence of antibodies to liver fluke in human blood by immunoelectrophoresis was reported by Teodorovic *et al.* (1963). The patient was a 9-year-old boy from Southern Yugoslavia, where human fascioliasis is described as common. One precipitation arch was seen in the γ-globulin region and is attributed to the antibody.

Test for Schistosomiasis?

It has been noted (p. 172) that liver-fluke antigens cross-react with antisera to *Schistosoma*. Mayer and Pifano (1944) thought of utilizing this reaction for diagnostic purposes in human populations; they envisaged using liver fluke antigen for intradermal tests so as to detect sufferers from *Schistosoma* infections. The practical advantage would be that liver fluke antigen is easier to obtain in large quantities. However, in a test on 133 persons, only half the bilharziasis sufferers gave a positive reaction to fluke antigen; and in every case the reaction was weaker than with *Schistosoma* antigen.

Workers repeating the experiments more recently have been similarly disappointed. Eliakim and Davies (1954) concluded that although the sera from patients with schistosomiasis may react with liver-fluke antigen, the titer is so low that the reaction is of no diagnostic value. Other workers attempted to pre-sensitize the skin of non-reacting persons with serum from positively reacting individuals. Again it was concluded that, although some cross reactions undoubtedly occur, they are neither constant nor strong enough to be useful in practice (Guerra *et al.*, 1945; Pautrizel *et al.*, 1962).

Note: The following additional references also include information about the course of fascioliasis in man: Abénte–Haedo *et al.* (1960); Galuez–Fermín (1948); Grote (1955).

PART IV

ECOLOGY AND CONTROL

CHAPTER 19

BIOLOGY OF THE SNAIL HOST

Habitat

Mozley (1957) described the locations in farmland where the snail is likely to occur and drew special attention to parts of fields where the turf has been trampled by hooves or wheels, to troughs, drains and ditches (except when covered over with thick grass), to shallow depressions in pasture etc. The snail may be carried by permanent streams, but does not stay there; nevertheless, it does not move very far from the water (Peters, 1938). It may be found in the algal mat often left on the ground by a recent flood.

It has been suggested that the distribution of the snail may be governed by the pH of the soil. The pH range favoured is given variously as 6–9 (Schadin, 1937), 6·2–7·2 (Mehl, 1932; Bryant, 1935). After examination of 22 farms and locations in Wales, Peters (1938) concluded that the snail prefers clay soil; the important factor may be soil impermeability to water rather than pH (Schmid, 1934). The role of the soil was illustrated by several workers. In Norway, the snail appears to favour quaternary clay (Ökland, 1935). In the valley of the North Rhine fascioliasis is present on the right shores of the river where the soils are clay and loamy, but is rare on the hilly and loess areas on the left of the river (Wetzel, 1953).

Location also affects the level of infestation of the snails with liver-fluke larvae, as was shown by a study in the Ukraine (Zdun, 1956): the proportion of infected snails was 2 per cent in the forest, 5 per cent in the steppe and 11 per cent in the mountains and foothills.

The presence of the snail host is not necessarily associated with the prevalence of the liver fluke. In Finmark (Norway) for example, *Limnaea truncatula* is present but fascioliasis is rare (Ökland, 1934). In the U.S.A., despite the favourable conditions for the snail hosts all along the Eastern seaboard, the liver fluke has so far established itself only in Florida, although it is abundant in Louisiana, Texas, California, Oregon, Washington, Nevada, Idaho, Utah and Montana; and also present, though rarer, in Arizona, New Mexico, Colorado, Arkansas, Wyoming, Michigan, Wisconsin, Alabama and Missouri (Price, 1953). The American snail host, *Stagnicola bulimoides techella* is restricted to soils of pH 7·1–8·4 (Olsen, 1944).

Life Cycle

At 9°C the snails hatch from their eggs in one month, at 17–19°C in 17–22 days and at 25°C in only 8–12 days (Roberts, 1950); they require a further 6–7 months to mature. Eggs are laid in the spring or in August–September (Schmid, 1934). In the laboratory, under favourable conditions 21 days suffice for the young snails to reach 0·5 cm in size and to start laying eggs. Egg-laying lasts for several weeks with one egg mass produced per day under favourable conditions. The egg masses cannot survive over 37°C nor do they develop below 10°C (Kendall, 1949, 1953).

Mehl (1932) found that the snail can survive dry conditions for 4 months, but in the laboratory this limit is not reached (Roberts, 1950). In greater detail, Kendall (1949) established that half-grown snails (0·3–0·5 cm) can survive for 1 yr, provided they aestivate with the shell opening sealed by apposition to the ground to prevent drying; no operculum is formed, despite a claim to the contrary by Rees (1932).

Predators of the Snail

It is not being suggested that predators are a likely means of effective control of the snail; but it may be of interest to note the observations that pleurodele newts eat snails (Fain, 1951), and that the snail may harbour in its mantle cavity an annelid worm, *Chaetogaster limnaei*, which seems to feed on the parasitic cercaria. Backlund (1949) found up to 10 worms per snail collected near Lund (Sweden) in October 1948 and each of these had up to 25 cercaria in its gut. Khalil (1961) was frustrated in his attempts to infect *Limnaea* because this worm consumed the larvae. Isoda *et al.* (1958) noted that carp feed on *Limnaea*. Michelson (1957) has collected all reports of predators and parasites of freshwater mollusca.

The Maintenance of Snail Colonies in the Laboratory

We owe to Taylor and Mozley (1948) a practical and efficient method of maintaining cultures of *Limnaea truncatula* (Appendix I). Such cultures are used for testing molluscicides and for maintaining a supply of liver fluke larvae for research.

N

CHAPTER 20

MOLLUSCICIDES

THE most widely used compound for the control of snails is copper sulphate (first used by Chandler, 1920), but its economical and effective application is not a simple matter. It is sprayed as a 5 per cent solution onto the soil or alternatively is dissolved in streams at the source (from where it seeps throughout the wet ground) and in ponds or ditches. It does not kill the eggs of the snail.

Copper sulphate need be applied only to the areas preferred by the snail; usually these areas occupy a small part of a farm.

A sufficiently high concentration must be maintained for some time before the compound acts. But high concentrations carry some risk. To mention one instance, Gracey and Todd (1960) reported chronic copper poisoning of sheep in Northern Ireland after grazing for a few weeks on pasture which had been sprayed three weeks earlier (September 1959) with 1 per cent copper sulphate. A level of 60–220 ppm of copper in the herbage dry matter persisted up to February, i.e. five months after spraying; it fell to 15–20 ppm (i.e. slightly over the level of unsprayed pasture) by May 1960 with the new season's growth of grass. Retention was helped by the dryness of the autumn in 1959. Dimercaptopropanol (B.A.L.) did not hasten excretion of the metal by the animals.

In locations where water seeps from a small stream Mozley (1957) recommended a precipitation method: Crystals of sodium carbonate are placed at some high point in the brook, and copper sulphate powder is immediately sprayed onto the area of seepage lower down. As the carbonate dissolves and reaches the lower area it precipitates the copper (as copper carbonate) in the form of particles that adhere to soil and grass and seep into recesses.

Even without the carbonate, copper sulphate applied at the source of a stream in amounts of 1 kg/50 l./min flow results in a high concentration (up to 1:500) in the upper section. In lower parts, a concentration of a thousand less may be maintained for days under favourable conditions, but edges and meanders must also be sprayed.

In still waters, an initial concentration of 1:100,000 need not be exceeded, especially as the compound tends to form a sediment and become absorbed on the bottom. If a 10 per cent hydrochloric acid is added to the spray this sedimentation tendency is reduced, thereby allowing more economical use of the copper (Tolgyesi, 1958).

Lungu and co-workers (1959) treated 45-hectare zones of different geo-climatic conditions. A 10 per cent concentrate in the form of aerosol (or in the case of low vegetation a 4–8 $\%_{000}$ spray) killed over 90 per cent of the snails, except in places with vegetation higher than 20 cm where efficiency was only 75 per cent. On the basis of their tests, these workers recommended the use of motor pumps for larger areas; for small streams, the placing of copper sulphate bags in the water; for puddles, direct spraying. Where there is a series of terraces, drains can be used to lead the solution from one to the next; high vegetation (over 30 cm) should first be cut. These workers also estimated that in Rumania only about 10 per cent of the total area of a given pasture requires treatment, on the average.

Sodium pentachlorophenate has also been tested both in the laboratory and the field (Enigk, 1958; Jordan et al., 1959). The former worker recommended a 5 per cent spray applied on wet ground or in rainy weather. This kills 100 per cent of *Limnaea truncatula* in 4 days. Other snails are even more sensitive:

mg/litre required for 100 *per cent kill in* 4 *days*

Limnaea ovata	1
Limnaea stagnalis	4
Planorbis cornutus	14
Planorbis planorbis	18
Vivipara vivipara	50
Fish (for comparison)	1

Australian workers have applied this compound (by dusting and spraying) against the local snail host of the liver fluke. They used 10 lb in 400 gallons of water per acre, after marking the snail habitat and cutting down high vegetation, but before draining. In their experience this compound is preferable to copper sulphate; furthermore, if ingested at the rate of up to 4 g per sheep it has no toxic effects.

Many other compounds have been tested. Comparing ammonium sulphate, potassium chloride, calcium superphosphate, ammonium nitrate and sodium nitrate, Vasileva (1960) found that only the ammonium nitrate has appreciable effects against *L. truncatula* in the laboratory. A 0·1 per cent concentration kills all snails within 48 hr, 0·2 per cent within 12 hr. However, in the field efficiency is much lower (73 per cent on swampy ground). But 0·4 per cent on swampy soil killed 94 per cent of the snails in 6 hr. The suggestion has been made that calcium cyanamide be used both as a fertiliser of pastures and a molluscicide, although this was considered impractical for areas irrigated with running water (Penso and Vianello, 1937).

The following compounds also have been tested: tetraethyl-monothiophosphate, tetraethyldithiophosphate (Funnikova, 1959). Under laboratory conditions 0·1 per cent of the first kills all snails within 5 days, 0·2 per cent within 42 hr. The second has the same results but with a longer delay. Three or more litres of the 0·2 per cent solution per hectare give an 85–100 per cent kill within 3 days, with snails in boxes placed on the ground. Under natural conditions an 81 per cent kill could be obtained within 8 days with a 1:1000 aqueous emulsion. The snails involved in these tests in Russia were *Limnaea stagnalis, Galba palustris* and *Radix lagotis,* the latter proving the most vulnerable of the three.

Another 135 compounds were screened against the snail hosts in Florida (*Pseudosuccinea columella* and *Fossaria cubensis*) under laboratory conditions. Copper sulphate bis (3-bromo-5-chloro-2-hydroxyphenyl) methane, and dinitro-o-cyclohexylphenol were the most effective. All snails exposed to them at a concentration of 1:800,000 for 24 hr and then transferred to fresh water eventually died, and all eggs failed to hatch. Wetting agents increased the effectiveness of the treatment. (Batte *et al.,* 1951 a and b; Batte and Swanson, 1952; 1962.)

CHAPTER 21

THE CONTROL OF FASCIOLIASIS

ATTEMPTS to control fascioliasis in a farm — or larger area — have two aims. Firstly to treat animals that have been exposed to risk, so as to improve their condition and to reduce the numbers of eggs discharged in the pastures. Secondly, to prevent new infections as far as possible. The first aim is served by dosing stock with a suitable anthelminthic; the second involves measures to reduce the snail population (molluscicides and drainage), and to keep stock away from risky locations, at least in the most dangerous periods (grazing management).

Weather and Snail Numbers — Forecasting

It has long been realised that weather conditions are the crucial factor in the enormous fluctuations of snail numbers from year to year. Furthermore (as explained in previous chapters) weather conditions affect the free larval stages of the fluke directly.

However, complete understanding of the correlation between weather conditions and the level of liver fluke infestation, to the point where it has predictive value, was achieved only by thorough investigations, such as those successfully carried out by workers at the Weybridge Veterinary Laboratory (see Ollerenshaw, 1958 a and b; Ollerenshaw and Rowlands, 1959; Ollerenshaw, 1959).

Anglesey was the first area to be studied, and the testing ground for the theory of forecasting; subsequently the theory has been verified elsewhere as well, and is now used for practical purposes on a large scale by the Ministry of Agriculture in the United Kingdom.

Fifty degrees F is a critical temperature, because at or below it the fluke larvae fail to develop; as a result, in Britain, development of eggs and larvae is suspended in late autumn, winter and early spring.

Within the remaining period of the year (May to October) the main factor governing growth of the snails is moisture. This affects activity, feeding and reproduction of the snail and thus determines the abundance of the parasitic larvae and the supply of cercaria. Also, moisture is necessary for the survival of the miracidia and cercaria themselves.

Development from the eggs to cercaria requires about 10 weeks, and the building up of cercarial numbers 12 weeks; it takes 14 weeks for the infestation of herbage to reach the highest level. Waterlogging of "flukey" areas, and indeed extension of these, occurs when rainfall exceeds evaporation during the reproductive

TABLE 20. FASCIOLIASIS IN NORTHERN IRELAND.
NUMBERS OF LIVERS CONDEMNED ON INSPECTION AT ABATTOIRS.

	1955*		1960		1962	
	Cattle	Sheep	Cattle	Sheep	Cattle	Sheep
Total kill	56,604	84,409	75,406	302,735	142,372	524,032
Condemned livers	37,931	19,336	51,832	33,352	90,844	62,678
Percentage condemned	67	22·9	68·7	11	63·8	12
Range between abattoirs	27·4– 94·3%		23·9– 93·8%	0·7– 31·2%	12·6– 88·6%	0·6– 33·2%
* Sheep by age: adult		55·7%				
lambs		12·8%				

Data supplied by Dr. J. F. Gracey (Gracey, 1961 and Annual Reports). The figures for 1955 and 1960 do not include the Belfast abattoir. For data per abattoir, see Fig. 62).

period. If and where such conditions last for 3 months within the May-to-October period, a heavy "flukey" year can be predicted.

Conditions of this type only rarely prevail in S.E. and E. England, but in hilly areas of the British Isles, with high rainfall, they are the rule (Fig. 62). However, the flukey areas or patches

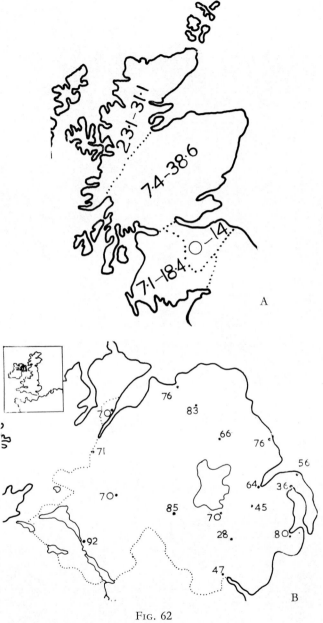

Fig. 62

in these districts are rather circumscribed because the soils are generally peaty and leached (acid and deficient in minerals); therefore they cannot support snails.

The most dangerous areas are therefore the lowlands with good soil and wet summers, as found in West England, Ireland (Table 20), and Wales, Anglesey being a typical example. October and September here are nearly always "wet", and this results in outbreaks of liver rot towards the end of October. Furthermore, many larvae are able to over-winter in the snail and if May and June of the following year are also wet months, a dangerous level of infestation of herbage is reached once again, with losses of farm animals from fascioliasis in August and September.

Thus two waves of cercaria and two peaks of infection may be expected in a year. The "summer infection" is the result of miracidia entering the snails in the summer and producing cercaria about 14 weeks later, i.e. late in the same season or autumn. The cysts will subsequently be picked up by stock and acute cases will appear from the autumn onwards (Fig. 63).

The "winter infection" is due to snails infected so late in the summer that larval development is interrupted by the winter, and completed in the spring, resulting in the early infection of pastures, and leading to the first acute cases of the summer.

Control Measures

Dosing

To decide on the best time for dosing, the conditions of development of the parasite in the current year should be reviewed, so as to give the carbon tetrachloride (or hexachlorethane) before large numbers of eggs have been discharged on the pasture.

FIG. 62. A. The percentage of "young" (first figure) and "old" second figure) sheep found to be infected with *Fasciola hepatica* in the four main regions of Scotland. The survey was carried out by examining 440 livers from 80 hill-sheep farms in the period 1946 to 1954 (Parnell *et al.,* 1954). "Young sheep" under 14 months old; "old sheep" over 14 months. B. The percentage of infected livers in cattle slaughtered at various abattoirs in Northern Ireland. The figures are averages of 1955, 1960 and 1962. (Data compiled by Dr. J. F. Gracey, see also Table 20.)

Acute cases of fascioliasis indicate the presence of younger flukes in the liver in large numbers, and should be the sign for undertaking the dosing of sheep. The acute cases should be given a heavier dose, 5 ml of carbon tetrachloride, because this dose is effective not only against any flukes in the bile ducts but also kills younger parasites down to 5–6 weeks old; the other animals should be given 1 ml.

Snail Control

The first step towards snail control is the identification of the fields or patches of ground where the snail host is found. This renders unnecessary the expensive and impractical indiscriminate spraying with copper sulphate solution.

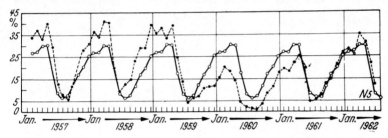

FIG. 63.   Percentage of condemned livers of lambs in six export abattoirs in Holland (Honer and Vink, 1963). The period covered is from January, 1957, to June, 1962.
Open circle line: Overall averages for each month throughout the period. Black dots line: Actual percentages for each year and month. The differences from the overall average are attributed by the authors cited to differences in weather conditions.

The molluscicide is best applied when the cercaria are about to leave the snail.

Where practicable, drainage would bring about a permanent reduction of snail numbers, as moisture favours the multiplication of the snail.

Grazing Management

Small flukey patches can be fenced so as to keep the grazing animals away. In the case of whole flukey fields, stock should be kept away from them at least during the period of the greatest load of cysts on the pasture, i.e. from September to spring.

Frequent change of pasture also helps reduce the infection of young lambs following their mothers.

The success of control measures presupposes the existence of a specialist service able to assess risks and to decide on recommendations based on the current conditions. But it also presupposes the readiness of farmers to apply these recommendations thoroughly. That this cannot always be taken for granted was shown in a survey of measures taken in about 100 farms in Anglesey and Cornwall during the 1958–59 epidemic (Ollerenshaw and Rowcliffe, 1961).

CONCLUSION

THE elucidation of the complex life history of *Fasciola hepatica* has been described as a landmark in the history of parasitology. But the biology of the parasite, with its polymorphic larval stages, still holds important secrets from the point of view of embryology, whilst its physiology remains largely unknown.

The recent development of suitable media and methods for maintaining the adult liver fluke *in vitro* in good condition for reasonable periods, has now made controlled physiological experimentation possible. Such physiological studies are particularly important because they are both directly and indirectly relevant to the problem of control of the liver fluke. For example, research on the probable passage of metabolites, including drugs, through the worm's body surface and their subsequent metabolism in its tissues might provide rational clues to improved chemotherapy.

At present, the chemotherapy of fascioliasis is meeting with a basic obstacle: the available drugs affect the adult flukes but leave intact the younger migratory stages. Large-scale screening of likely compounds is continuing and should produce better drugs. Eventually, these combined with the diagnostic tests that have been developed by immunological investigation, might provide means for more radical treatment of affected stock.

Apart from giving rise to several useful diagnostic tests, the work on the immunology of fascioliasis has so far met with a paradoxical situation. Mammals produce antibodies, but these antibodies impart no clear-cut or lasting protection from subsequent infection.

Obviously, research will now be directed at discovering the reasons for this ineffectiveness of antibodies. The work so far does not seem to provide any clue as to possible causes, and research workers will have to check as many likely hypotheses as possible. Is it that the antibodies are kept at elbow-length from the parasite's tissues simply by the worm eating up at a high rate the antibody with the liver tissue? Or do the antibodies actually reach the surface of the parasite but become inactivated by it? Would antibodies to antigens collected not from adult flukes but from metacercaria prove more effective against the migratory stages?

The prevention of infection will always remain an important part of the effort for keeping fascioliasis in check. Ecological studies have proved their value in this respect; they have led to the accurate delineation of the conditions favouring the parasite and its snail host; they have thus made possible the identification of the infested regions or even locations within single farms and explained the distribution of the disease. What is more important, they have produced a method of forecasting the severity of future outbreaks, thus greatly facilitating the economical organization of control work. Measures for the reduction of the snail population, whether by drainage or by molluscicides, or for the reduction of mammalian infections by appropriate pasture management, all owe their development to ecological research.

Further work in this sector may indicate new practical ways of reducing the risk to farm animals: for example, by restricting infested locations to the production of silage rather than grazing, as the metacercarial cysts do not survive the process of silage production. The role of alternative "reservoir" hosts of the parasite should also be studied.

As none of the separate approaches, ecological, immunological or chemotherapeutic, has by itself led to an easy solution to the problem of fascioliasis, farmers have to rely in the meantime on planned control campaigns integrating several methods — such as chemotherapy, diagnostic tests, pasture management and drainage. There is no doubt that such campaigns are effective (as has been shown repeatedly) and that they can strikingly reduce the size of the problem. But it is hoped that research will eventually result in more economical and more radical methods of control of the liver fluke, by means of a drug or a vaccine.

THE HANDLING OF LIVER FLUKE MATERIAL

1. Eggs, Embryonation and Hatching of Miracidia

Eggs may be obtained from the bile, or from live worms collected from the bile ducts of infected liver. Also, of course, they may be separated from the faeces of infected animals (see 2).

To remove eggs from adult flukes, rinse the worms and dissect and open the uterus under a binocular. Select mature eggs, i.e. those that are already yellow and sink to the bottom of the petri dish.

Embryonic development will require about 7 days if the eggs are kept in the incubator at 27°C, and 6–8 weeks at 16°C; eggs can be stored (in distilled water) in the refrigerator for about a month before being transferred to the incubator.

The eggs must be washed, and the water changed daily and shaken to keep bacteria and protozoa down and to separate eggs clumping together. Let the beaker stand for 10 min to allow eggs to settle to the bottom before draining off the water down to the last half-inch. To reduce clumping spread the water with the eggs, after washing, in the petri dish where they are kept.

After 7 days transfer the eggs to a more or less dark refrigerator for about 3 days. When movement of miracidia is seen in the first few eggs, keep the lot in absolute darkness at 4°C if you wish to prevent the miracidia from hatching. They can last for a month in this state.

To induce hatching, transfer embryonated eggs to watch-glass and add some fresh distilled water. Mass hatching should follow in 5–10 min and can be observed under the microscope; the heat from the microscope light helps (Eales, 1930; Jepps, 1933; Rowan, 1956).

2. Egg Counting in Faeces

Nearly 100 per cent recovery of eggs from the faecal sample is required for counts in a haemocytometer. But this is not important when only confirmation of fascioliasis is the aim.

Simplified procedures for separating eggs from faeces are given below:

(a) *Precipitation Technique* (Carballeira *et al.*, 1959)

Collect faecal samples: plastic bags are suitable.

Disperse 200 g of the sample in half its volume of water.

Homogenize as finely as possible.

Pass through a 10 mesh per cm² filter, into 1000 ml of water, and let settle for at least 5 min.

Remove and reject the top 700 ml.

Pass the remaining 300 ml through a 20/cm² mesh, into 1000 ml of water and let settle.

Remove the top 800 ml.

Repeat twice again.

Collect the precipitate and examine for eggs under microscope.

(b) *A Flotation Procedure* (Teuscher, 1957)

Weigh 2·5 g of faeces.

Disperse the sample in 37·5 ml of water.

Filter through a 1 mm mesh.

Mix the filtrate well with an equal amount of the following flotation solution:

$$\begin{matrix} 80 \text{ g zinc sulphate} \\ 25 \text{ g sugar} \end{matrix} \quad \text{in 100 ml of water).}$$

Let the mixture stand 6–8 hr.

Examine the top layer for eggs.

(c) *Formol-Ether Precipitation Technique* (Ridley and Hawgood, 1956; used for the Detection of Human Fascioliasis by Facey and Marsden, 1960).

Weigh 1·0 g of faeces.

Emulsify the sample in 7 ml of 10 per cent formol saline.

Strain through a wire gauze (40 mesh to the inch) into a centrifuge tube.

Add 3 ml of ether and shake vigorously for 1 min.

Centrifuge, accelerating gradually over a period of 2 min to 2000 rpm.

Switch centrifuge off and let it come to rest.

Loosen from the wall of the tube the debris on the surface and at the interphase of the two liquids; decant the supernatant allowing the last 1–2 drops to run back.

Wipe the outer part of the tube clean of debris, shake up the small deposit and pour into the haemocytometer.

3. Maintenance of a Snail Culture — Cysts

The snail, *Limnaea truncatula,* can be bred in the laboratory for experimental purposes. The techniques required have been developed mainly by Kendall (1953), and are of course modified in practice by individual workers. At the same time a continuous culture of algae for feeding the snail must be maintained.

Algal Culture

The algae are cultured in glass or earthenware dishes as follows:

1. Collect clay topsoil; sterilize it by dry heat or autoclave for at least 30 min at 160°C, in order to free it of worms, seeds etc.

2. Soak the soil in distilled water, let it cool, and soak again until it becomes soft. Remove stones and other objects, and work it by hand to a soft and pliable mud.

3. Transfer enough soil to dishes to cover bottom to a thickness of 1 in.; smooth the surface with moistened fingers.

4. Transfer (by spatula or finger) some fresh green algae from mud in a locality where liver fluke abounds. A mixed culture of algae, with *Oscillatoria sp.* predominating, is used in many laboratories. Smooth the algae evenly into the soil with some slight pressure. About one hour later cover the surface of the soil with a shallow layer of distilled water.

5. Keep the dishes covered with glass, and under strong light, but avoid too much heat, say over 27°C. Replenish the water, keeping the algae just covered with it. A rich growth of algae, giving off gas bubbles, will have formed in less than a week. After this, the dishes should be removed from the strong light and used within a week.

Snails

The snails are placed a few in each algal dish and left until they eliminate the algal covering of the soil.

When about 1 month old they lay egg-masses; they may live for about a year, and breed continuously in the laboratory. Transfer the egg masses onto damp filter paper in covered Petri dishes. The young should hatch in 2–3 weeks. Just before hatching the egg masses are transferred to new algal dishes.

Note that when snails are placed in an algal dish, enough water should be left in it to form a small "pool" at the centre.

Infection of Snails with Miracidia

Young snails (a few weeks old) are placed in glass tubes with a little distilled water, after the shell is cleaned of mud. A few hatched miracidia are transferred by pipette into the tube.

After 5 hr or more, when penetration will be complete, the snails may be transferred to algal pans.

Emergence of Cercaria

About 9 weeks after infection, and at two-week intervals after that, masses of cercaria may be obtained from the snails. It should be understood that liver fluke cysts can infect man and animals and this operation should not be undertaken where there are no facilities for sterilizing glassware etc.

Transfer a snail into a watch-glass or preferably a tube, and wash it with a fine jet of water, avoiding contamination of hands, benches etc.; transfer clean snail to a tube, cover it with cork and place at a temperature of about 12°C for 1–1·5 hr.

Now raise temperature slowly to room temperature and leave for several hours or a whole day, by which time the cercaria will have encysted on the tube wall.

The cysts can be kept in a refrigerator (preferably after the water in the tubes has been changed), for a month or more.

Infection of Mammal

The cysts can be dislodged from the wall of the tube by careful scraping and given to mammals by pipette through the mouth, or in gelatine capsules.

4. Hatching of Cysts (Wikerhauser, 1960)

Prepare two enzyme solutions: (a) Pepsin (0·5 g of pepsin and 0·8 g of sodium chloride in 100 ml of N/20 hydrochloric acid), and (b) Trypsin (0·4 g of trypsin, 0·8 g of sodium chloride and 1 g of $NaHCO_3$ in 100 ml of water). The metacercaria are left in the first solution for 2–3 hr and this partly digests the outer layer of the cyst; the cyst becomes transparent so that the occasional movements of the larva in it can be seen. However, no excystment follows until the trypsin solution is also poured in, when within another 2–3 hr the metacercaria become active and eventually excyst. A high rate of excystation (80 per cent) is induced by the addition of 20 per cent of ox bile to the solution.

Whilst the excysted metacercaria are themselves digested after 2 hr in the above medium, they can survive for up to 42 hr in Tyrode's saline solution (with penicillin and streptomycin added).

5.   Examination of Adult Liver Flukes

As mentioned, adult liver flukes may be collected from the bile ducts of infested livers; it might be possible to obtain such a liver fresh from the local abattoir. The flukes can be washed in ordinary saline if there is no intention of keeping them alive for long.

Examinations possible on the live adult worm include visualizing the gut or the excretory system by injection of a vital dye (such as Evan's blue) in solution in saline. A fine glass pipette is made by drawing out the finest available glass tubing in a flame. The pipette is connected to a length of rubber tubing. For the insertion of the pipette end through the oral sucker a binocular is required; the fluke is transferred onto a glass slide and the sucker is manipulated with a forceps. Once the pipette end is inserted, the dye solution is blown gently out of the pipette. It will be seen that the solution spreads from the more anterior to the more posterior caeca and to their branches. If the pipette is pushed further in, it may get into the excretory bladder and the dye solution will spread from there not into the gut but into the excretory tubules (Fig. 33). The dye soon fades and spreads, hence the specimen should be examined immediately, kept flat between two slides.

Regarding histology, the liver fluke presents no special problems of fixation. Any general fixative may be used. However, Flemming's fixative retains and stains the fat droplets which (in section) show up the course of the excretory tubules (Fig. 34).

Visualization of Yolk Glands. Staining Reactions of Egg-Shell Material

These reactions have been studied by Smyth (1951, 1954) and Johri and Smyth (1956). The first paper deals with the staining

o

reactions of egg-shell granules in the yolk and gives details for staining these (with methyl-green pyronin or malachite green). The staining shows up the whole yolk gland system.

The 1956 paper deals with other staining reactions of the phenolic compounds contained in the yolk. It is from these phenolic compounds that quinone is formed (enzymatically) in the presence of oxygen. The quinone in turn interacts with protein in the egg-shell material, resulting in tanning or change of the protein to sclerotin. After this has occurred, exposure to air will turn the egg-shell brown. The stain used here (Fast Red) will tint the yolk glands yellow or orange to red.

However, a better technique for the visualization of yolk glands in whole mounts is given in the 1954 paper (Fig. 47). The enzyme transforming diphenol to quinone (polyphenol oxidase) can also form quinone from catechol. As the automatic tanning of material is very slow in the liver fluke, Smyth adds catechol, and the quinone formed from this then gives rise to sclerotin quickly. Because of the large amount of eggs and of egg-shell material so affected the whole vitelline system is emphasized clearly in whole mounts.

The procedure given is as follows:
(1) Fix the whole fluke in 70 per cent alcohol — 24 hr.
(2) Wash in water — 30 min.
(3) Incubate in 0·2 per cent. Catechol (Analar, freshly prepared same day) — 30–90 min.
(4) Wash in water — 30 min.
(5) Dehydrate in 70 per cent, 90 per cent and absolute alcohol.
(6) Pass through xylene and mount in Canada balsam.

6. *In Vitro* Maintenance of Liver Flukes

The flukes must be removed from the bile ducts under nearly aseptic conditions, and special solutions must be available. An incubator and some simple tissue culture equipment are required. For details and references see Chapter 14.

PREPARATION AND FRACTIONATION OF LIVER-FLUKE ANTIGENS

THE procedures used by various authors cited in the text are given here for two reasons. Firstly, the reader may wish to compare the details of the techniques used. Secondly, the description of these procedures would be particularly useful to research workers wishing to investigate the immunology of fascioliasis further.

1. Preparation of "Antigen" for Skin Tests

Fasciola hepatica, adult flukes
Wash in saline; incise to wash out caecal contents
Dry at 37°C for 4 days
Powder in sterile mortar
Store at −10°C

Suspend in saline (100 ml/g)	Suspend in absolute alcohol (100 ml/g)
Leave for 10 days at 4°C	Leave for 24 hr at 37°C
Centrifuge	Filter
Sterilize the clear supernatant at 56°C for 45 min.	Concentrate until precipitate appears (to about ⅓ of volume)
Centrifuge	Increase volume with alcohol to 50 ml (precipitate redissolves)
Store in rubber-sealed bottles at −10°C	Store in rubber-sealed bottles
(Trawinski, 1959)	(Lavier and Stefanopoulo, 1944) These authors remark that the alcoholic suspension keeps better, although a saline suspension is also active.

2. Preparation of Protein Antigen (Urquhart *et al.,* 1954)

Fasciola hepatica, adult flukes.
Wash in tap water.
Suspend in 1 ml of 0·9 per cent NaCl per worm.

Homogenize.

Let it stand at 0–4°C for several hours to let large particles settle.

Collect the supernatant.

Centrifuge insoluble material out at 3000 rpm for 1 hr.

(The saline extract so obtained is usually amber to dark brown and contains 1 mg of protein nitrogen per ml).

For Alum Preparations

Treat the extract from the above treatment with an equal volume of 10 per cent w/v of potash alum.

Adjust pH to 6·5 with 5N NaOH.

Collect precipitate and wash it twice with 0·9 per cent NaCl (containing 1:1,000,000 merthiolate).

Suspend in 0·9 per cent NaCl (merthiolated) for injection.

The use of alum has the purpose of increasing the potency of antigens. Formula of alum: $AlCl_3 \, 6H_2O$.

Kjehldahl analyses have shown that the above procedure precipitates the same amount of protein Nitrogen as 10 per cent TCA (trichloracetic acid). In other words the alum precipitate contains all the protein in the saline extract.

For More Purified Precipitating Antigen

The saline extract is salt-fractionated as follows:

(a) Half-saturate with ammonium sulphate; collect the precipitating protein fraction; repeat. Use the precipitate as the precipitating antigen.

(b) Treat the saline extract with 1 vol. of saturated ammonium sulphate and stir.

Let solution stand at 0–4°C for several hours.

Collect the precipitate by centrifugation.

Treat the precipitate with 1 vol. of 0·1 phosphate buffer of pH 8.

Remove materials that do not redissolve, by centrifuging.

Precipitate a protein fraction by the procedure under (a).

Dialyse the precipitate against 0·9 per cent NaCl until the dialysate gives no reaction with Nessler's reagent.

(At each precipitation and during dialysis there is some loss of protein as insoluble residue and the yield ultimately obtained is usually about 10 per cent of the total protein in the original extract).

3. Preparation of Antigen (Ershov, 1959, and Collaborators)

Fasciola hepatica, adult flukes.

Wash.

Weigh.

Homogenize.

Suspend in three volumes of water or saline.

Add the enzyme pancreatin (7–10 g/l.), sodium bicarbonate (10–15 g/l.) and chloroform (10 ml/l).

Maintain pH at 7·4–8·2 by adding bicarbonate when pH drops to acid;

without lifting cork, shake every 1–2 hr. Keep in incubator at 38–40°C (for up to 3 days for the process of digestion to be completed, by which time the emulsion becomes clear; only the eggs remain undigested).
Collect supernatant and centrifuge it at 2000 rpm for 3–5 min.
Add five volumes of 96 per cent alcohol.
Leave 24 hr, by which time the flaky precipitate collects (this precipitate is described as a stable complex of the antigen).
Collect the precipitate and dry it *in vacuo* or thermostat.

N.B. The complex is essentially a polysaccharide of glucose and glucosamine (not glycogen) linked with peptides. The polysaccharide represents 60 per cent and the protein 30–40 per cent. The complex has a very low toxicity, 200 mg being required to kill a mouse in a day.

4. Purification of Antigen by Maekawa (1954)

	Fasciola hepatica, adult flukes
	Homogenize in 10 vol. of water
	Boil for 30 min at 100°.
	Supernatant
(Fraction I)	Saturate with $(NH_4)_2 SO_4$
Precipitate	Supernatant
	Extract with 5 vol. of 90 per cent phenol
	Extract
	Add alcohol to 10 per cent
	Supernatant
	Add alcohol to 85 per cent; adjust pH to 5·6
Precipitate	Supernatant
	(Fraction II)
	Extract with NH_4OH (pH 8·5) five times more by weight
	Extract
	Adjust pH to 4·4
	Supernatant
	Add alcohol to 85 per cent; adjust pH to 5·6
Precipitate	Supernatant
	(Fraction III)
	Dissolve in 0·1 N acetic acid, 10:1 by volume
Precipitate	Extract
	Adjust alcohol to 56 per cent; adjust pH to 4·4
	Supernatant
(Fraction IV)	Add alcohol to 85 per cent; adjust pH to 5·6
Precipitate	Supernatant
	Dissolve in 40 vol. of water
	Add acetone to 67 per cent
	Supernatant
	Dialyse; adjust pH to 4·4; lyophylise; wash with acetone to 65 per cent; centrifuge
	Crystalline Fraction V

5. Electrophoretic Separation

Biguet, Capron and Tran Van Ky (1962) prepared an extract in 0·018 M
NaCl from liver flukes homogenised in the cold. The extract was separated
from the tissue debris by centrifugation for 1 hr at 12000 rpm, and was then
dialysed and frozen-dried. When this "standard antigen" was subjected to
electrophoresis on starch gel in Poulik's discontinuous buffer it gave rise to
13 protein bands (Fig. 64).

Antiserum was obtained from rabbits that were given for about 4 months
one injection a week of crude fluke homogenate mixed with Freund's
incomplete adjuvant. This antiserum and the "standard antigen" were used
for immunoelectrophoresis on agar gel, and gave rise to 15 reaction curves;
some of these however were not specific to the liver fluke but appeared also
with extracts from certain other helminths. The order of appearance of
these 15 antibody fractions is shown in Fig. 61.

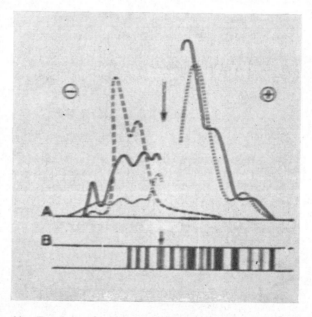

Fig. 64.   Fractions of rabbit antibody to the liver fluke, as separated
by starch gel electrophoresis (Biguet, Capron and Tran Van Ky, 1962).
The arrow indicates the origin, where the serum sample was inserted,
the vertical bands represent diagrammatically the protein fractions as
stained by Amido-Black. The graphs show the densities of the various
fractions. Continuous line, all fractions stained by Amido-Black.
Interrupted line, glycoprotein fractions stained by PAS. Dotted line,
lipoprotein fractions as stained by Sudan Black. + anode. − cathode.

REFERENCES

ABENTE-HAEDO, F., RODRIGUEZ-DEVINCENZI, A. M., OSIMANI, J. J. and NESCIA, W. (1960) Un brote epidémico en Florida de Distomatosis humana por *Fasciola hepatica*. *An. Fac. Med. Montevideo*, **45**, 319–329.

AGERSBORG, H. P. K. (1924) Studies on the effect of parasitism upon the tissues. I. with special reference to certain gastropod molluscs. *Quart. J. micr. Sci.*, **68**, 361–401.

ALBISTON, H. E. (1927) Infectious necrotic hepatitis of sheep in Victoria. A braxy-like sheep disease. *Aust. J. exp. Biol. med. Sci.*, **4**, 113–123.

ALICATA, J. E. (1953a) Human fascioliasis in the Hawaiian Islands. *Hawaii Med. J.*, **12**, 196–201.

ALICATA, J. E. (1953b) The snails, *Pseudosuccinla columella* (Say), new intermediate hosts for the liver fluke *Fasciola gigantica* Cobbold. *J. Parasit.*, **39**, 673–674.

ALVARADO, R. (1949) Sur la structure histologique de *Fasciola hepatica*. 13ème Congrès International de Zoologie (1948) 450–451.

ALVARADO, R. (1951a) El tegumento, la musculature y el parénquima de *Fasciola hepatica*. *Trab. Inst. Cienc. nat. Acosta*, **3**, 1–90.

ALVARADO, R. (1951) El epitelio cuticular de las vías genitales de *Fasciola hepatica*. *Bol. soc. esp. Hist. nat.*, **49**, 159–162.

ANDRAŠKO, M. (1959) Skuzenosti zjarnej odčervovacej akcie novadzieno dobytka v prešovskoi kraji. *Veterinářstvi, Brno*, **9**, 455–456.

ANDREEV, A. I. (1953) Fascioliasis in pigs and its treatment. *Veterinariya*, **30**, 26–27.

ANON. (1956) Liver flukes of sheep. *Rural Research in G.S.I.R.O., Melbourne*, No. 17, 11–16.

ANON. (1959) Liver fluke outbreak in Wales. *Vet. Rec.*, **71**, 57.

BABENSKAS, M., PAGIRYS, J. and ALISAUSKAITE, V. (1958) (Diagnosis of fascioliasis in farm animals and methods for its control in the Lithuanian S.S.R.). *Acta parasit. lithuanica*, **1**, 121–133.

BACIGALUPO, J. (1932) *Limnea viatrix* d'Orb infectée par des cercaires de *Fasciola hepatica* á Buenos Aires. *C.R. Soc. Biol.*, **111**, 828.

BACIGALUPO, J. (1933) Superposition geographique de *Fasciola hepatica* L. et de *Limnaea viatrix* d'Orb. *C. R. Soc. Biol.*, **112**, 492–493.

BACIGALUPO, J. (1934) La evolución de la *Fasciola hepatica* en la Republica Argentina. *Actas y Trab., Congresso Nac. Med.*, **3**, 950–956.

BACKLUND, H. O. (1949) En kommensal som äter sit värddjurs parasiter. *Fauna o. Flora*, **44**, 38–41.

BACQ, Z. M. and OURY, A. (1937) Note sur la repartition de la cholinestérase chez les êtres vivants. *Acad. Roy. Belg. Bull. Classe des Sciences*, **23**, 891–893.

208 REFERENCES

BARKE, A. (1958) Untersuchungen zum antihelminthischen Wirkungs-mechanismus des Piperazin. *Dtsch. tierärztl. Wschr.*, **65**, 65–68.

BASNUEVO, J. G. (1954) Fascioliasis hepatica tratada con cloroquine y emetina. *Rev. Med. trop., Habana*, **10**, 79–80.

BASNUEVO, J. G. (1955) Cloroquina y emetina intramuscular en el tratamiento de la amibiasis, la fascioliasis y la clonoschiasis. *Rev. Med. trop., Habana*, **11**, 5–8.

BATTE, E. G. and SWANSON, L. E. (1950) Control of the common liver fluke in cattle. *Rep. Fla agric. Exp. Sta.*, Year 1949–50, 105–106.

BATTE, E. G. and SWANSON, L. E. (1952) Liver fluke control and its relation to snail ecology, *Proc. Am. Vet. Med. Assoc.*, **88**, 101–105.

BATTE, E. G. and SWANSON, L. E. (1952b) Laboratory evaluation of organic compounds as molluscicides. *J. Parasit.*, **38**, 65–68.

BATTE, E. G., Swanson, L. E. and MURPHY, J. B. (1951a) Control of fresh-water snails (intermediate hosts of liver flukes) in Florida. *J. Am. Vet. Med. Assoc.*, **68**, 139–141.

BATTE, E. G., SWANSON, L. E. and MURPHY, J. B. (1951b) New molluscicides for the control of fresh-water snails. *Am. J. Vet. Res.*, **12**, 158–160.

BECEJAC, S. and LUI, A. (1959) O djelovanju teperature i kisika na razvoj jaja velikog metilja (*Fasciola hepatica* L.). *Veterin. Arkiv*, **29**, 293–301.

BEHRENS, H. (1960) Behandlung des Leberegelbefalls der Schafe mit Hetol. *Dtsch. Tierärztl. Wschr.*, **67**, 467–470.

BENEDEK, L. and NEMESERI, L. (1953) Die mikroskopische Diagnose der Leberegelseuche. *Acta vet. hung.*, **3**, 415–422.

BÉNEX, J., LAMY, L. and GLEDEL, J. (1959) Etude de la réaction de fixation du complément à l'antigen distomien chez le mouton. *Bull. Soc. Pat. expt.*, **52**, 83–87.

BERTHIER, L. (1954) Contribution à l'étude du tégument de *Fasciola hepatica* L. *Arch. Zool. exper. gen.*, **91** (NR), 89–102.

BETTANCOURT, A. and BORGES, I. (1922) Réaction de fixation dans la citharziose vésicale avec antigène de *Fasciola hepatica*. *C. R. Soi. de Biol.*, **136**, 1053.

BETTENDORF, H. (1897) Über Muskulatur und Sinneszellen der Tremato-den. *Zool. Jahrb. Abt. Anat.*, **10**, 307–358.

BHALERAO, G. D. (1933) The Trematode parasites of the Indian elephant, *Elephas indicus. Indian J. veter. Sci. anim. Husb.*, **3**, 103–115.

BIAGI, F. F., TAY, J. and PORTILLA, J. (1958) Valor de una intradermo-reaccion de precipitacion en el diagnostico de la fasciolosis humana. *Rev. Lat. Amer. Microbiol., Mexico*, **1**, 69–78.

BIDLOO, G. Brief van G. Bidloo aan Anthony van Leeuwenhoek, vvegens de dieren, welke men zomtyds in de lever der schaapen en andere beesten vind. H. van Kroonevelt, Delft, 1698.

BIGGART, J. H. (1937) Human infestation with *Fasciola hepatica*. *J. Path. Bact.*, **44**, 488–9.

BIGUET, J., CAPRON, A. and PH. TRAN VAN KY (1962) Les antigènes de *Fasciola hepatica*. *Ann. Paras. hum. comp.*, **37**, 221–231.

BJÖRKMAN, N., THORSELL, W. and LIENERT, E. (1963) Studies on the action of some enzymes on the cuticle of *Fasciola hepatica* L. *Experientia*, **19**, 3–5.

BJÖRKMAN, N. and THORSELL, W. (1962) The fine morphology of the mitochondria from the parenchymal cells in the liver fluke (*Fasciola hepatica*, L.). *Exp. Cell. Res.*, **27**, 342–346.

BJÖRKMAN, N. and THORSELL, W. (1964) On the fine structure and resorptive function of the cuticle of the liver fluke, *Fasciola hepatica* L. *Exp. Cell Res.*, **33**, 319–329.

BOGOMOLOVA, N. A. (1956) The role of nucleic acids in the oogenesis and fertilization of *Fasciola hepatica*. *Dokl. Acad. Nauk SSSR*, **110**, 461–464.

BOGOMOLOVA, N. A. (1957a) Cytochemical examination of the miracidium of *Fasciola hepatica* L. *Dokl. Acad. Nauk SSSR*, **117**, 313–315.

BOGOMOLOVA, N. A. (1957b) A cytological study of the miracidium of *Fasciola hepatica* L. *Dokl. Akad Nauk SSSR*, **117**, 942–944.

BOGOMOLOVA, N. A. (1961) *Radix ovata* as one of the intermediate hosts of *Fasciola hepatica*. *Zoolog. Shurnal*, **40**, 774–775.

BOJANUS, L. H. (1818) *Kurze Nachricht über die Zerkarien und ihren Fundort.* Isis von Oken, Jahrg., 729–730.

BONCIU, C., POP, A., HEITMANEK, C., RASMEVITA, C., LESCINSKY, S. and MARGINEANU, A. (1954) Contributii la studiul leziunilov produse de *Fasciola hepatica* la cobai. *Studdii si Cercetări de Luframicobiologie, Bucharest*, **5**, 505–514.

BORAY, J. C. and PEARSON, I. G. (1960) The anthelminthic efficiency of tetrachloro difluoroethane in sheep infected with *Fasciola hepatica*. *Aust. Vet. J.* **30**, 331–337.

BORAY, J. C. and MCMICHAEL, D. F. (1961) The identity of the Australian Lymnaeid snail host of *Fasciola hepatica* and its response to environment. *Austr. J. Mar. Freshw. Res.*, **12**, 150–163.

BORCHERT, A. (1954) Ermittlung parasitärer Krankheiten durch die Kotuntersuchung. *Mh. Vet. Med.*, **9**, 38–39.

BOSHAN, C. J., THOROLD, P. W. and PURCHASE, H. S. (1961) Investigation into the development of hexachlorophene as an anthelminthic. *J. S. Afr. Vet. Med. Ass.*, **32**, 227–233.

BOVIEN, P. (1931) Notes on the cercaria of the liver fluke (*cercaria Fasciolae hepaticae*). *Vidensk. Medd. dansk. naturh. Foren. Kbh.*, **92**, 223–226.

BRAND, T. VON (1928) Beitrag zur Kenntniss der Zusammensetzung des Fettes von *Fasciola hepatica*. *Zschr. Vergl. Physiol.*, **8**, 613–624.

BRAND, T. VON and MERCADO, T. I. (1961) Histochemical glycogen studies on *Fasciola hepatica*. *J. Parasit.*, **47**, 459–463.

BRAND, T. VON and WEINLAND, E. (1924) Über tröpchenförmige Ausscheidungen bei *Fasciola hepatica*. *Z. wiss. Biol.*, C, **2**, 209–214.

BRAUN, M. *Digenea.* In Brönn's *Klassen und Ordnungen des Thierreichs*, Bd. 4, Abteil. Ia, 566–925, Leipzig, 1879–93.

BREMNER, K. C. (1961) The copper status of some helminth parasites with particular reference to host-helminth relationships in the gastro-intestinal tract of cattle. *Austr. J. agric. Res.*, **12**, 1188–1199.

BROCQ-ROUSSEAU, CAUCHEMEZ, L. and URBAIN, A. (1923) La réaction de déviation du complément appliqué au diagnostic de la distomatose ovine. *Bull. Soc. Cent. Med. vet.*, **124**, 54.

BRODY, T. M. (1959) Mechanism of action of carbon tetrachloride. *Fed. Proc.*, 1017–1019.

BRYANT, A. (1935) An experimental investigation into the pH range of various species of *Limnaea*. *Proc. Liverpool Biol. Soc.*, **49**, 8–16.

BRYANT, C. and SMITH, M. J. H. (1963) Some aspects of intermediary metabolism in *Fasciola hepatica* and *Polycelis nigra*. *Comp. Biochem. Physiol.*, **9**, 189–194.

BRYANT, C. and WILLIAMS, J. P. G. (1962) Some aspects of the metabolism of the liver fluke, *Fasciola hepatica* L. *Exp. Paras.*, **12**, 372–376.

BUGGE, G. (1927a) Über die Veränderungen der Lungen und der Pleura des Rindes durch *Fasciola hepatica*. *Dtsch. Tierärztl. Wschr.*, **35**, 133–135.

BUGGE, G. (1927b) Zur Entwicklung der *Fasciola hepatica*. I. Entwicklung des Darmes. *Dtsch. Tierärztl. Wschr.*, **35**, 575–581 and 594–596.

BUGGE, G. (1927c) Vergleichende Untersuchungen über die Distomatose bei Rindern und bei Schafen. *Tierärztl. Rdsch.*, **33**, 833–838.

BUGGE, G. (1928) Über den Invasionsweg der *Fasciola hepatica* ber der Distomatose der Rinder und Schafe. *Berl. Tierärztl. Wschr.*, **44**, 189–195.

BUGGE, G. (1929) Beginnt das Excretionsgefässystem der *Fasciola hepatica* mit terminalorganen? *Berl. tierärztl. Wschr.*, **45**, 557–561.

BUGGE, G. (1935) Die Wanderungen der Leberegel in den Organen der Schlachttiere, *Berl. tierärztl. Wschr.*, **101**, 65–68.

BUGGE, G. and MÜLLER, G. H. (1928) Zur Ursache der hepatitis interstitialis multiplex des Schweines (Distomatose). *Berl. Tierärztl. Wschr.*, **44**, 293–296.

BÜHNER, F. and PFEIFER, K. (1960) Ein neues Mittel für die Therapie des Befalles der Schafe mit dem grossen Leberegel (*Fasciola hepatica*). *Mh. Vet. Med.*, **15**, 400–404.

BÜHNER, F. (1961) Weitere Erfahrungen über die parenterale Leberegeltherapie insbesondere die koprologische und klinische Kontrolle der Ursodistolwirkung. *Mh. Vet. Med.*, **16**, 140–142.

BUTLER, J. B. and HUMPHRIES, A. (1932) On the cultivation in artificial media of *Catenaria anguillulae*, a Chytridiacean parasite of the ova of the liver fluke, *Fasciola hepatica*. *Sci. Proc. R.Dublin Soc.*, **20** (NS), 301–304.

BUTLER, J. B. and BUCKLEY, J. J. C. (1927) *Catenaria anguillulae* as a parasite of the ova of *Fasciola hepatica*. *Sci. Proc. R. Dublin Soc.* (NS), **18**, 497–512.

BUTOZAN, V., TOMIC, L. and HORVATIC, I. (1961) Uloga anaerobne infekcije (a Welchii tip. A) u akutnoj metiljavosti ovaca. *Veterinaria, Sarajevo*, **10**, 9–23.

BUTYANOV, D. D. and GUZMAN, Z. I. (1960) Comparison of the efficacy of difluorotetrachloroethane (Freon-112) and carbon tetrachloride against fascioliasis in sheep. *Trud. nauch.-issled. veter. Inst., Minsk*, **1**, 179–181.

BYLCHOWSKI, B. (1957) Monogenetitcheskie sosalchtiki ik sistema i philogenia. *Pub. Lab. Zool. Acad. Sc. URSS, Leningrad.*

CALLOT, J. and GAYOT, G. (1946) Etude expérimentale de la survie de *Fasciola hepatica. Rev. Med. Veter. Lyon-Toulouse*, **97**, 249–250.

CAMERON, T. W. M. (1951) *The parasites of domestic animals.* London.

CAMPBELL, W. C. (1957) *Fascioloides magna* (Trematoda), with special reference to the adult in relation to disease. *Dissertation Abstracts,* **17**, 2092.

CAMPBELL, W. C. (1961a) Nature and possible significance of the pigment in fascoloidiasis. *J. Parasit.,* **46**, 769–775.

CAMPBELL, W. C. (1961b) Notes on the egg and miracidium of *Fascioloides magna* (Trematoda). *Trans. Amer. Micr. Soc.,* **80**, 308–319.

CARBALLEIRA, D., BAUTISTA, A., VARELA, D., COMPAIRE, C., ROSON, R., FIERRO, D., PAREDES, L. and PLATERO, A. (1959). Una aportation al diagnóstico coprológico de la distomatosis hepática. *Report XVI Intern. Veter. Congress, Madrid,* **2**, 591–597.

CARRARA, O. and RECALCATI, M. (1961) Incidenza della distomatosi epatica nei bovini nazionali macellati in Provincia di Milano. *Soc. ital. Sci. veter.,* **15**, 542–545.

CATELLANI, G. (1952) Le alterazioni delle linfoghiandole bronchiali e mediastiniche nella distomatosi polmonare dei bovini. *Atti Soc. ital. Sci. vet.,* **6**, 284–289.

CHANCE, M. R. A. and MANSOUR, T. E. (1949) A kymographic study of the action of drugs on the liver fluke (*Fasciola hepatica*). *Brit. J. Pharmacol.,* **4**, 7–13.

CHANCE, M. R. A. and MANSOUR, T. (1953) A contribution to the pharmacology of movement of the liver fluke. *Brit. J. Pharm.,* **8**, 134–138.

CHANDLER, A. C. (1920) Control of fluke diseases by destruction of the intermediate host. *J. agric. Res. U.S. Dept. Agric.,* **20**, 193–208.

CHANDRASEKHARIAH, H. R. (1951) Fascioliasis in buffaloes. *Indian vet. J.,* **27**, 457–458.

CIELESZKY, V. and KOVÁCS, F. (1958) Szarvasmarhák széntetrakloridos kegelésének hatása a tejre es tejtermèkekre. *Magyar. Allatorv. Lapja,* **13**, 279–281.

CLAISSE, R. and HARTMARK, L. (1954) Caractères biologiques, sérologiques et histologiques de la distomatose hépatique. *Arch. Mal. Appar. dig.,* **43**, 197–205.

CLEGG, J. A. (1957) Studies on the maintenance of *Fasciola hepatica in vitro.* Ph.D., thesis, University of London.

COE, W. R. (1896) Notizen über den Bau des Embryos von *Distomum hepaticum. Zool. Jahrb., Anat. u. Ontog.,* **9**, 561–570.

CONDOS, A. C. and MCCLYMONT, G. L. (1961) Pharmacology and toxicology of carbon tetrachloride in the sheep. I. Blood levels following ruminal, abomasal and intramuscular administration. *Aust. J. agr. Res.,* **12**, 433–439.

CONDOS, A. C., SOUTHCOTT, W. H. and McCLYMONT, G. L. (1963) The toxic and anthelminthic effects in intraruminal and intramuscular injections of CCl₄ in the sheep. *Aust. J. agr. Res.,* **14,** 852–866.

CONDY, J. B. (1962) Fascioliasis — a disease of major economic importance. *Rhod. agric. J.,* **59,** 259–262.

CORT, W. W., AMEEL, D. J. and VAN DER WOUDE, A. (1948) Studies on germinal development in rediae of the Trematode order Fasciolatoidea Szidat, 1936. *J. Parasit.,* **34,** 428–451.

CORT, W. W., AMEEL, D. J. and VAN DER WOUDE, A. (1954) Parasitological Reviews. Germinal development in the sporocysts and rediae of the digenetic Trematodes. *Exp. Parasit.,* **3,** 185–226.

COUDERT, J. (1952) Remarques sur le diagnostic parasitologique, et les critères de quérison de la distomatose hépatique à l'homme. *Lyon Med.,* **33,** 565–568.

COUDERT, J. and GARIN, J. P. (1959) Essais de traitement de la distomatose hépatique de l'homme par la 4–7 phenanthroline-5-6 quinone. *Lyon Med.,* **91,** 527–530.

COYLE, T. J. (1956) Liver fluke in Uganda. *Bulletin of Epizootic Diseases in Africa,* **4,** 47–55.

CULBERTSON, J. T. and TALBOT, S. B. (1935) A new antagonistic property of normal serums: the cercaricidal action. *Science,* **82,** 525.

CURASSON, G. (1931) Recherches sur la diagnostic des distomatoses à *Fasciola hepatica* et *Amphistomum cervi* par les réactions allergiques. *Bull. Acad. Vét. Fr.,* **8,** 77.

DAVTYAN, E. A. (1953) *Acute fascioliasis in sheep.* Izd. Akad. Nauk. S.S.S.R. (Moscow), 205–210.

DAVTYAN, E. A. (1956) Pathogenicity of different species of *Fasciola* and its variability depending on the developmental conditions of the parthogenetic stages. *Zool. Zhurnal,* **35,** 1617–1625.

DAWES, B. (1946) *The Trematoda.* Cambridge.

DAWES, B. (1954) Maintenance *in vitro* of *Fasciola hepatica. Nature,* **174,** 654–655.

DAWES, B. (1960) A study of the miracidium of *Fasciola hepatica,* and an account of the mode of penetration of the sporocyst into *Limnaea truncatula.* Libro-homenaje Dr. Caballero y Caballero, 95–111.

DAWES, B. (1960a) Penetration of the liver fluke, *Fasciola hepatica* into the snail, *Limnaea truncatula. Nature,* **185,** 51–52.

DAWES, B. (1960b) The penetration of *Fasciola hepatica* into *Limnaea truncatula* and of *F. gigantica* into *L. auricularia. Trans. R. Soc. trop. Med. Hyg.,* **54,** 9–10.

DAWES, B. (1961a) On the early stages of *Fasciola hepatica* penetrating into the liver of an experimental host; the mouse; a histological picture. *J. Helminth.,* Leiper Suppl., 41–52.

DAWES, B. (1961b) Juvenile stages of *Fasciola hepatica* in the liver of the mouse. *Nature,* **190,** (477b), 646–647.

Dawes, B. (1962a) On the growth and maturation of *Fasciola hepatica* L. in the mouse. *J. Helminth,* **36,** 11–38.

Dawes, B. (1962b) Additional notes on the growth of *Fasciola hepatica* L. in the mouse — with some remarks about recent researches in Belgium. *J. Helminth,* **36,** 259–268.

Dawes, B. (1962c) A histological study of the caecal epithelium of *Fasciola hepatica* L. *Parasitology,* **52,** 483–493.

Dawes, B. (1963a) The migrating of juvenile forms of *Fasciola hepatica* L. through the wall of the intestines in the mouse, with some observations on food and feeding. *Parasitology,* **53,** 109–122.

Dawes, B. (1963b) Some observations of *Fasciola hepatica* L. during feeding operations in the hepatic parenchyma of the mouse, with notes on the nature of liver damage in this host. *Parasitology,* **53,** 135–144.

Dawes, B. (1963c) Hyperplasia of the bile duct in fascioliasis and its relation to the problem of nutrition in the liver-fluke. *Parasitology,* **53,** 123–134.

Dawes, B. and Müller, R. (1957). Maintenance *in vitro* of *Haplometra cylindracea. Nature,* **180,** 1217.

de Jesus, Z. (1935) *Lymnaea philippinensis,* an intermediate host of *Fasciola hepatica* in the Philippines with some observations on the bionomics of the parasite. *Philipp. J. Sci.,* **58,** 299.

Dennis, W. R., Stone, W. M. and Swanson, L. E. (1954) A new laboratory and field diagnostic test for fluke ova in faeces. *J. Am. Vet. Med. Assoc.,* **124,** 47–50.

Demidov, N. V. (1953). *Subcutaneous application of carbon tetrachloride for fascioliasis in sheep.* Izd. Akad. Nauk. SSSR. (Moscow), 226–233.

Demidov, N. V. (1954) Treatment of *Fasciola* infection in sheep with carbon tetrachloride. *Veterinariya,* **31,** 16–18.

Demidov, N. V. (1955) *Difluorotetrachlorethane* and *filixan* in fascioliasis in sheep. *Veterinariya,* **32,** 29–32.

Demidov, N. V. (1958) Further investigations with difluorotetrachloro-ethane against fascioliasis in cattle. *Byull. Inst. Gelmintologii im. Akadem. Skryabina,* **4,** 36–38.

Demidov, N. V. (1959) Chemotherapy of Fascioliasis. *Byull. Inst. Gelmintologii im Skryabina.* No. 5, 25–29.

Demidov, N. V. and Veselova, T. P. (1959) Treatment of fascioliasis in cattle. *Veterinariya,* **36,** 12–13.

Deron, E., Meirsman, J. L., Landsheere, B. C. and Derom, F. (1956) Extraction d'une grande douve vivante de cholédoque chez un malade atteint de lithiase biliaire et d'ictère hémolytique familial. Premier observation belge de distomatose humaine par F. H. *Acta gastro-ent. belg.,* **19,** 219–229.

Deschiens, R. (1958) Les distomatoses hépatiques humaines en France. *Ann. Inst. Pasteur Paris,* **94,** 256–271.

Deschiens, R. and Poirier, M. (1950) L'intoxication expérimentale du cobaye par l'extrait de *Fasciola hepatica. C. R. Soc. Biol., Paris,* **144,** 1345–1346.

DESCHIENS, R. and POIRIER, M. (1953) Etude comparée des propriétés toxiques et éosinophilogènes de différent extraits de douves chez le cobaye. *C. R. Soc. Biol., Paris,* **147,** 1059–1061.

DESCHIENS, R. and BÉNEX, J. (1960a) Etude du sérum sanguin dans les bilharzioses humaines. *C. R. Acad. Sci., Paris,* **251,** 2103–2104.

DESCHIENS, R. and BÉNEX, J. (1960b) Etude électrophorétique de sérum sanguin dans la distomatose hépatique humaine. *C. R. Acad. Sci.,* **250,** 1380–1381.

DINNIK, J. A. and DINNIK, N. N. (1956) Observations on the succession of redial generations of *Fasciola gigantica* Cobbold in a snail host. *Z. Tropenmed. u. Parasit.,* **7,** 397–419.

DINNIK, J. A. and DINNIK, N. N. (1956) Systematics, distribution and life-histories of stomach flukes. *Rep. E. Afr. Vet. Res. Org.* (1955–56), 35–39.

DINNIK, J. A. and DINNIK, N. N. (1959) Effects of the seasonal variations of temperature on the development of *Fasciola gigantica* eggs in Kenya Highlands. *Bulletin of Epizootic Diseases of Africa,* **7,** 357–369.

DINNIK, J. A. and DINNIK, N. N. (1961) On the morphology and life-history of *Fasciola Nyanzae,* Leiper, 1910, from the hippopotamus. *J. Helminth,* R. T. Leiper, Suppl., 53–62.

DISSHMARN, R. (1955) La douve du foie, du bœuf et du buffle en Thailande. *Bull. Off. int. Epiz.,* **43,** 435–438.

DODD, S. (1918b) Studies in black disease. A braxy-like disease of sheep. *J. comp. Path.,* **31,** 1–35.

DODD, S. (1921) The etiology of black disease: Being further studies in a braxy-like disease of sheep. *J. comp. Path.,* **34,** 1–26.

DORSMAN, W. (1956a) New technique for counting *Fasciola hepatica* eggs in cattle faeces. *J. Helminth.,* **30,** 165–172.

DORSMAN, W. (1956b) Fluctuation within a day in the liver fluke egg — count of the rectal contents of cattle. *Vet. Rec.,* **68,** 571–574.

DORSMAN, W. (1959a) Hexachlorophen (G11) against liver fluke (*Fasciola hepatica*), in cattle. *Tijdschr. Diergeneesk.,* **84,** 100–103.

DORSMAN, W. (1959b) A new treatment of cattle against liver fluke, *Fasciola hepatica. Reports of* 16*th International Veterinary Congress,* Madrid, 1959, vol. 2, 609–612.

DOUGHERTY, J. W. (1952) Intermediary protein metabolism in helminths. I. Transaminase reactions in *Fasciola hepatica. Exp. Parasit.,* **1,** 331–338.

DOUGHERTY, J. W. (1952) Studies on the protein metabolism of certain helminth parasites. *J. Parasit.,* **38,** (suppl.), p. 32.

DUKHOVSKOI, S. (1956) Subcutaneous injection of carbon tetrachloride for *Fasciola* infestation of sheep. *Veterinariya,* **33,** 45.

DURBIN, C. G. (1952) Longevity of the liver fluke, *Fasciola hepatica*, in sheep. *Proc. Helminth. Soc., Washington,* **19**, 120.

DYSON, F. L. (1959) Human fascioliasis (Correspondence). *Brit. med. J.,* **1**, 1301.

DZIEKÓNSKI, J. (1947) Badania nad ogniskami pasozytniczymi w wezlach Chlonnych lydla. *Méd. Vét.,* **3**, 140–142.

EALES, N. B. (1930) A method of obtaining stages in the life-history of the liver fluke for class purposes. *Nature,* **125**, 779.

EGOROV, L. F. (1954) Longevity of *Fasciola hepatica. Veterinariya,* **31**, 25.

EHRLICH, I., FOREMBACHER, S., RIJAVEC, M. and KURELAC, B. (1960a) Istraživanja o skutnoj metiljavosti. I. O mekim klinickim i biokemÿskim promjenama kod akutne metiljavosti goveda. *Vet. Arkiv.,* **30**, 229–236.

EHRLICH, I., FORENBACHER, S. RIJAVEC, M. and KURELAC, B. (1960b) Istraznanja o skutnoj metiljavosti. II. O utjecaju atebrina na migracioni stadij velikog metilja u organizmu goveda i o moquenostima lijecenja akutne metiljavosti atebrinom. *Vet. Arkiv.,* **30**, 307–313.

EHRLICH, I. and WINTERHALTER, M. (1958) O ulozi terapije klorinanim ugljikovodicina u plomskom suzbijanju fascioloze. *Vet. Glasnik,* **12**, 266–269.

EHRLICH, I., LUI, A. and WINTERHALTER, M. (1957) Djelovanje heksakloretana na lyečena goveda, metilje i njihova jaja. *Vet. Arkiv.,* **27**, 392–414.

EHRLICH, I., LUI, A. and WINTERHALTER, M. (1958) Über die fasciolocide und ovocide Wirkung des Tetrachlorkohlenstoffs (CCl₄) bei Schafen. *Dtsch. tierärztl. Wschr.,* **65**, 323–326.

ELIAKIM, M. and DAVIES, A. M. (1954) The complement fixation test in bilharziasis. I. The value of different extracts of *Schistosoma mansoni* and *Fasciola hepatica* worms as antigens. *Parasitology,* **44**, 407–413.

ENIGK, K. and DÜWEL, D. (1958) Zur Wirksamkeit des "Distan" beim Leberegelbefall. *Dtsch. tierärztl. Wschr.,* **65**, 240–242.

ENIGK, K. and DÜWEL, D. (1959) Zur Häufigkeit der pränatalen Infektion mit *Fasciola hepatica* beim Rinde. *Berl. Münch. Tierärztl. Wschr.,* **72**, 362–363.

ENIGK, K. (1958) Die Vernichtung von Süsswasser- und Landschnecken. *Ceskoslov. Parasit.,* **5**, 59–65.

ENIGK, K. and DÜWEL, D. (1960) Die Behandlung der fasciolose beim Rind mit Hetol-R. *Dtsch. tierärztliche Wschr.,* **67**, 537–539.

ERHARDOVÁ, B. (1961) Vývojový cyklus motolice obrovské *Fasciola magna* v podminkách ČSSR. *Zool. Listy, Brno.,* **10**, 9–16.

ERSHOV, V. S. (1959) The problem of immunization of domestic animals to helminthoses. *Reports of* 16*th International Veterinary Congress,* Madrid, 1959, vol. 1, 279–289.

FACEY, R. V. and MARSDEN, P. D. (1960) Fascioliasis in man: outbreak in Hampshire. *Brit. med. J.,* **2**, 619–625.

FAIGUENBAUM, J. (1958) Distomatosis hepatica humana con especial referencia a complicaciones quirurgicas. *Bol. chil. Parasit.,* **13**, 29–31.

216 REFERENCES

FAIGUENBAUM, J., AGOSIN, M. and TAMARGO, A. (1950) Distomatosis humana. *Rev. méd. Chile,* **78,** 384–387.

FAIGUENBAUM, J., VACCAREZA, A., JIMINEZ, E., HURTADO, R., D'ACUÑA, G. and APABLAZA, A. (1958). Distomatosis humana. Differentes modalidades clinicas observadas en cuatro casos. *Bol. chil. Parasit.,* **13,** 69–73.

FAIN, A. (1951) *Lymnaea (Radix) natalensis,* transmetteur naturel de *Fasciola gigantica* au Congo belge. Reproduction expérimentale du cycle évolutif de cette douve. *Ann. Soc. Belge Med. Trop.,* **31,** 531–539.

FAIN, A. (1951) Notes écologiques et parasitologiques sur *Lymnea (Galla) truncatula* Müller au Congo belge. *Ann. Soc. Belge Méd. trop.,* **31,** 149–152.

FAIRBURN, D. (1958) Trehalose and glucose in helminths and other Invertebrates. *Canad. J. Zool.,* **36,** 787–795.

FAUST, E. C. (1919) The excretory system in *Digenea. Biol. Bull.,* **36,** 315–344.

FAUST, E. C. (1920) Pathological changes in the gastropod liver produced by fluke infection. *Johns Hopkins Hosp. Bull.,* No. 31, 79–84.

FAUTREZ, J. (1958) Etude histochimique de l'oocyte de premier ordre. *C. R. Ass. Anat.,* **45,** 1.

FEDERMANN, M. (1959) Die Behandlung des Leberegelbefallens. *Dtsch. tierärztl. Wschr.,* **66,** 526–529.

FEDYUSHIN, V. P. and UTESHEV, A. I. (1952) Non-specific tubercular reactions in cattle with fascioliasis. *Veterinariya,* **29,** 32–35.

FLORKIN, M. and DUCHATEAU, G. (1943) Les formes du système enzymatique de l'uricolyse et l'évolution du catabolisme purique chez les animaux. *Arch. Intern. Physiol.,* **53,** 267–307.

FLURY, F. and LEEB, F. (1926) Zur Chemie und Toxikologie der Distomen (Leberegel). *Klin. Wochschr.,* **5,** 2054–2055.

FRAIPONT, J. (1880) Recherches sur l'appareil excréteur des Trématodes et des Cestodes. I. *Arch. Biol., Gand.,* **1,** 415–456.

FRAIPONT, J. (1881) Recherches sur l'appareil excréteur des Trématodes et des Cestodes. II. *Arch. Biol., Gand.,* **2,** 1–40

FRENKEL, H. S. (1907) Distomatosis hepatis suis. *Zschr. f. Infekt. Krh. der Haust.,* **2,** 546–549.

FRIEDL, F. E. (1960) Induced hatching of operculate eggs. *J. Parasit.,* **46,** 454.

FRIEDL, F. E. (1961a) Studies on larval *Fascioloides magna.* I. Observations on the survival of rediae *in vitro. J. Parasit.,* **47,** 71–75.

FRIEDL, F. E. (1961b) Studies on larval *Fascioloides magna.* II. *In vitro* survival of axenic rediae in amino acids and sugars. *J. Parasit.,* **47,** 244–247.

FRIEDL, F. E. (1961c) Studies on larval *Fascioloides magna.* IV. Chromatographic analysis of free amino acids in the haemolymph of a host snail. *J. Parasit.,* **47,** 773–776.

FROYD, G. (1960) The incidence of liver flukes (*Fasciola gigantica*) and hydatid cysts (*Echinococcus granulosus*) in Kenya cattle. *J. Parasit.,* **46,** 659–662.

FUNNIKOVA, S. V. (1959) Testing of organic phosphorus compounds for the control of molluscs. *Trudi Kazansk. Veterinarn. Inst.,* **13,** 387–397.

GÁLLEGO-BERENGUER, J. (1952) Un caso de teratologia en trematodes. Atrofia unilateral total de la glandula vitelogena en *Fasciola hepatica*. *Rev. iber. Parasit.*, **12**, 65–67.

GÁLVEZ FERMÍN, N. (1948) Fascioliasis del coledoco. (Reporte de un caso operado). *Rev. Med. trop. Habana*, **4**, 191–192.

GANASEVICH, V. I. and SKOVRONSKI, R. V. (1956) Treatment of rabbits against fascioliasis. Problemi Parazitologii (Transactions of the 2nd scientific conference of parasitologists of the Ukranian SSR).

GARIPUY, A., DASTE, B., GOUZI, G. and MALLARET, P. (1953) Distomatose duodénale à *Fasciola hepatica*. *Maroc méd.*, **32**, 614–616.

GASKELL, J. F. (1914) The chromaffine system of Annelids and the relation of this system to the contractile vascular system in the leech, *Hirudo medicinalis*. *Phil. Trans. Roy. Soc. Lond.*, **205**, 53–211.

GAUSE, G. F. and SMARAGDOVA, N. P. (1940) The decrease in weight and mortality in dextral and sinistral individuals of the snail, *Fruticicola lautzi*. *Amer. Nat.*, **74**, 568–570.

GAVEL, I. I., KRESAN, A. S. and GONCHARUK, E. G. (1958) Subcutaneous application of carbon tetrachloride against fascioliasis in sheep. *Veterinariya*, **35**, 81.

GAVRILYUK, P. Y. (1956) Intramuscular injection of carbon tetrachloride for *Fasciola* in sheep. *Veterinariya*, **33**, 45.

GEBAUER, O. (1958) Kalk und seine Beziehungen zur Leberegelbekämpfung. Vorläufige Mitteilung. *Arch. exper. Veterinärmed.*, **12**, 79–81.

GEBAUER, O. (1958) Die Untersuchung von Schweinelebern auf das Vorkommen von Leberegeln. *Wien. Tierärztl. Mschr.*, **45**, 659–660.

GIAMPORCARO, S. and BIANCO, A. (1955) Contributo alla diagnosi delle distomatosi canina applicazione pratica di una nuova tecnica per l'esame coprologico. *Profilassi*, **28**, 88–92.

GINETSINSKAYA, T. A. (1960) The relationship between the distribution of glycogen in the bodies of different cercariae and their biological peculiarities. *Dokl. Akad. Nauk. SSSR.*, **135**, 949–951.

GINETSINSKAYA, T. A. (1961) The dynamics of fat deposition in the life cycle of Trematodes. *Dokl. Akad. Nauk. SSSR.*, **139**, 1016–1019.

GIORDANO, A. (1959) Il midollo osseo nella distomatosi dei Giovani Bufali. *Acta. Med. Vet., Naples,* **5**, 67–72.

GLÄSSER, K. (1949) Zur Bekämpfung der Rinder-Enteritis. *Dtsch. Tierärztl. Wschr.*, **56**, 373–374.

GLÄSSER, K. and WEITZNER, B. (1948) Nochmals die Distomatose des Rindes in ihrer Beziehung zu den Enteritisbakterienausscheidern und zum Kallerparatyphus. *Mh. Vet. Med.*, **3**, 151–152.

GODERDZISHVILI, G. I. (1955) Role of some species of fresh water snails in fascioliasis in the Leningrad region and the effects of some mineral fertilizers on them. *Leningrad. Inst. Usovershenst. Vet. Vrachei*, **10**, 219–223.

P

GOIL, M. M. (1958) Protein metabolism in trematode parasites. *J. Helminth,* **32,** 119–124.

GOIL, M. M. (1961) Haemoglobin in trematodes. I. *Fasciola gigantica.* II. *Cotylophoron indicum. Z. Parasitenk.,* **20,** 572–575.

GOIL, M. M. (1961) Physiological studies on trematodes — *Fasciola gigantica* carbohydrate metabolism. *Parasitology,* **51,** 335–338.

GOLDSCHMIDT, R. (1909) Eischale, Schalendrüse und Dotterzellen der Trematoden. *Zool. Anz.,* **34,** 481–489.

GOMES, F. and XAVIER, A. (1956) A proposito de un novo caso de fascioliase hepatica humana: ensaio sobre a tecnica de fixacao do complemento paradiagnostico serologicer. *Ann. Inst. Med. trop., Lisboa,* **13,** 901–910.

GOMULKIN, A. A. (1957) Needle puncture and the creation of fistulae of the gall bladder in the cow. *Sborn. Nauchn. Trud.,* No. 11, 185–191.

GONCHARUK, I. S. (1959a) Appearance and biochemical properties of meat from cattle infected with fascioliasis. *Sborn. nauch. Trud. Lovoski Zoovet. Inst.,* **9,** 203–211.

GONCHARUK, I. S. (1959b) Beef output from cattle infected with *Fasciola. Sborn. nauch. Lvovski Zoovet. Inst.,* **9,** 213–214.

GÖNNERT, R. (1962) Histologische Untersuchungen über den Feinbau der Eibildungsstätte (Oogenotop) von *Fasciola hepatica Zschr. Parasitenk.,* **21,** 475–492.

GOODCHILD, C. G. (1958) Implantation of *Schistosomatium doushitti* into the eyes of rats. *Exp. Parasit.,* **7,** 152–164.

GORDON, H. McL. (1955) Fascioliasis, referred to acute fluke disease. *Aust. vet. J.,* **31,** 46–47.

GORDON, H. McL. (1955) Some aspects of fascioliasis. *Aust. vet. J.,* **31,** 182–189.

GORDON, H. McL., PEARSON, I. G., THOMSON, B. J. and BORAY, J. G. (1959) Copper pentachlorphenate as a molluscicide for control of fascioliasis. *Aust. vet. J.,* **35,** 465–473.

GORYANOVA, E. S. (1957) The use of ruminography in the diagnosis of asymptomatic forms of fascioliasis. *Uchen. Zap. Vitebsk. Veter. Inst.,* **15,** 74–78.

GOVAERT, J. (1953a) Deoxyribonucleic acid content of the germinal vesicle of the ovocyte in *Fasciola hepatica. Nature,* **172,** 302–303.

GOVAERT, J. (1953b) Sur la teneur en acide désoxyribonucléique du noyau des cellules vitellogènes chez *Fasciola hepatica. C. R. Soc. Biol., Paris,* **147,** 1494–1496.

GOVAERT, J. (1954) La teneur en acide désoxyribonucléique des noyaux des éléments de la lignée spermatique chez *Fasciola hepatica. Biol. Jahrb.,* **21,** 202–209.

GOVAERT, J. (1955) Etude quantitative de l'acide désoxypentosenucléique lors de la maturation et de la fécondation de l'oeuf chez *Fasciola hepatica. C. R. Soc. Biol., Paris,* **149,** 1066–1069.

GOVAERT, J. (1960) Etude cytologique et cytochimique des cellules de la lignée germinative chez *Fasciola hepatica. Exp. Parasit.,* **9,** 141–158.

GRACEY, J. F. (1961) *Survey of Livestock Diseases in Northern Ireland.* London, H.M.S.O.

GRACEY, J. F. and TODD, J. R. (1960) Chronic copper poisoning in sheep following the use of copper sulphate as a molluscicide. *Brit. vet. J.,* **116,** 405.

GREGOIRE, C., POUPLARD, L., COTTELEER, C., SCHYNS, P., THOMAS, J. and DEBERDT, A. (1956) Nouvelle méthode de diagnostic. La distomatose. *Ann. Med. Veterinaire,* **100,** 294–303.

GREMBERGEN, G. VAN (1944) Le métabolisme respiratoire du cestode *Monesia benedeni. Enzymologia,* **11,** 268–281.

GREMBERGEN, G. VAN (1949) Le métabolisme respiratoire du trématode *Fasciola hepatica* Linn. *Enzymologia,* **13,** 241–257.

GREMBERGEN, G. VAN (1950) Au sujet de la nutrition chez *Fasciola hepatica. Ann. Soc. zool., Belge,* **81,** 15–20.

GRESSON, R. A. R. (1957) Spermatoleosis in *Fasciola hepatica. Quart. J. Micr. Sci.,* **98,** 493–498.

GRESSON, R. A. R. and THREADGOLD, L. T. (1959) A light and electron microscope study of the epithelial cells of the gut of *Fasciola hepatica* L. *J. bioph. bioch. Cytol.,* **6,** 157–162.

GRETILLAT, S. (1961) Note préliminaire sur l'épidemiologie de la distomatose bovine au Sénégal. *Rev. Elevage Med. vet. Pays Tropic,* **14,** 283–291.

GRIFFITHS, H. J. (1962) Fascioloidiasis of cattle, sheep and deer in Minnesota. *J. am. vet. Med. Ass.,* **140,** 342–347.

GRIGORYAN, G. A., KHANBEKYAN, R. A. and OVANESYAN, A. S. (1955) Treatment of fascioliasis in sheep with hexachlorethane and carbon tetrachloride. *Veterinariya,* **32,** 53–56.

GRIGORYAN, G. A. (1956) Influence of external environmental factors on the biology and resistance of miracidia and metacercariae of *Fasciola gigantica. Trudi Armyansk. Inst. Zhivotn. Veterin.,* **9,** 93–99.

GRIGORYAN, G. A. (1958) Experimental data on *Fasciola gigantica* infection of sheep. *Trudi Armyansk. Inst. Zhivotn. Veterin.,* **3,** 155–168.

GRIGORYAN, G. A. (1959) Experimental data on length of survival of the adolescariae of *Fasciola gigantica. Veterinariya,* **36,** 35–37.

GROTE, K. (1955) Fasciolosis als Ursache einer Hepatosplenomegalie. *Mschr. Kinderheilk.,* **103,** 482–484.

GUERRA, P., MAYER, M. and DiPRISCO, J. (1945) La especifidad de las intra-dermoreacciones con antigenos de Schistosoma mansoni y *Fasciola hepatica* por el metodo de Prausnitz-Kuestner. *Rev. Sanid. y Assist. Soc. Caracas,* **10,** 51–63.

GUNST, J. A. and MANEN, A. VAN (1948) Onderzoek naar het voorkomen van paratyphus bacillen in de gal en tevens van de kiemhoudendheid van de gal lij normale bedrijfsslachtingen van runderen. *Tijdschr. voor Diergeneesk.,* **73,** 103–106.

GÜRALP, N. (1954) ICI firmasiniu yeui biv anthelmentik ilaci "Minel" ile yaptigimiz deneyler ve alddigimir sonuclar. *Türk. vet. Hekim. dern. Derg.*, **24**, 1597–1604.

GÜRALP, N. and SIMMS, B. T. (1959) Bionomics of *Fasciola hepatica* in Turkey. *Vet. Fak. Yaginl.*, **6**, 173–183.

HABERKERN, W. (1951) Die Darmflora des Schafes mit besonderer Berücksichtigung der Verteilung des *Bacterium coli* in verschiedenen Darmabschnitten und die Bedeutung der Leberegelkrankheit bei Schafen. Dissertation, Munich, 1951.

HARNISCH, O. (1932a) Untersuchungen über den Gaswechsel von *Fasciola hepatica*. *Z. wiss. Biol.*, **17C**, 364–386.

HAVET, J. (1900) Contribution a l'étude du système nerveux des Trématodes (*Distomum hepaticum*), *La Cellule*, **17**, 353–381.

HAY, J. (1949) Obserwacje nad intensywnoscia jajeczkawania motylicy watrobowej w ciagu calego roku. *Méd. vét., Varsovie*, **5**, 171–178.

HEALY, G. R. (1955a) Studies on immunity to *Fasciola hepatica* in rabbit. *J. Parasit.*, **41**, 25.

HEALY, G. R. (1955b) Anomalies in *Fasciola hepatica*. *J. Parasit.*, **41**, 35.

HEIDA, Y. (1956) Distomatose-bestrijding door middel van capsules tetrachloorkoolstof. *Tijdschr. Diergeneesk.*, **81**, 1019–1024.

HEIN, W. (1904) Zur Epithelfrage der Trematoden. *Zschr. f. Zool.*, **77**, 546–585.

HENDELBERG, J. (1962) Paired flagella and nucleus migration in the spermiogenesis of Dicrocoelium and Fasciola (Digenea, Trematoda). *Zool. Bidrag, Uppsala*, **35**, 569–587.

HENNEGUY, L. F. (1902) Sur la formation de l'œuf, la maturation et la fécondation de l'oocyte chez *Distomum hepaticum*. *C. R. Acad. Sci.*, **134**, 1235–1238.

HENNEGUY, L. F. (1906) Recherches sur la mode de formation de l'oeuf ectolécithe du *Distomum hepaticum*. *Arch. Anat. micr.*, **9**, 47–88.

HEVIA, H., SCHENONE, H., KLEIN, O. and ALARCON, R. (1958) Distomatosis cutanea asociada a erupcion reptante. *Bol. chil. Parasit.*, **13**, 57–59.

HIGASHI, T. (1960a) Infection mechanisms of helminths and pathological studies on the effects of intestinal microorganisms. Relationship of *B. subtilis* and a mechanism of infection with *Fasciola hepatica*. I. Parasitological observations on guinea pigs. *Jap. J. Parasit.*, **9**, 470–479.

HIGASHI, T. (1960b) Infection mechanism of helminths and pathological studies on the effect of intestinal microorganisms. II. Pathological observations on guinea pigs. *Jap. J. Parasit.*, **9**, 673–684.

HOFFMAN, W. A. (1930) The intermediate host of *Fasciola hepatica* in Puerto Rico. *Puerto Rico J. publ. Hlth trop. Med.*, **6**, 89–90.

HONER, M. R. and VINK, L. A. (1963) Contributions to the epidemiology of fascioliasis hepatica in the Netherlands. I. Studies on the dynamics of fascioliasis in lambs. *Z. f. Parasitenk.*, **22**, 292–302.

HÖPPLI, R. (1921) Die Diagnose pathogener Trematoden durch Blutuntersuchung. *Arch. Schiffs u. Tropenhyg.*, **25**, 365.

HORSTMANN, H. J. (1962) Sauerstoffverbrauch und Glycogengehalt der Eier von Fasciola hepatica während der Entwicklung der Miracidien. *Zschr. Parasitenk.*, **21**, 437–445.

HOVE, E. L. (1949) Comparison of fatal tocopherol deficiency disease in rats with the syndrome caused by CCl_4. *Ann. N. Y. Acad. Sci.*, **52**, 217–224.

HUBENDICK B. (1951) Recent Lymnaeidae. Their variation, morphology, taxonomy, nomenclature and distribution. *Kungl. Svenska Vetenskapsakademiens Handlingar,* Fjärde Serien, Band 3, No. 1.

HUGHES, D. L. (1962) Reduction of the pathogenicity of *Fasciola hepatica* in mice by irradiation. *Nature, (Lond.),* **193**, 1093–1094.

HUGHES, D. L. (1963) Some studies on the host–parasite relations of *Fasciola hepatica.* Ph.D. Thesis, University of London.

HUGHES, D. L. (1959) Chemotherapy of experimental *Fasciola hepatica* infections. M.Sc. Thesis, University of London.

IBROVIC, M. and GALL-PALLA, V. (1959) Meka klinička patološko-anatomska i biohemiska zapažanja u vezi s okutnom masovnam metiljavošcu ovaca. *Veterinariya, Sarajevo,* **8**, 531–537.

ICHIHARA, T., SUSUMI, S. and KURAMOTO, T. (1956) Studies on the diagnosis of fascioliasis. I. Antigens for the precipitation test. *Jap. J. vet. Sci.,* **18**, 119–129; **18**, 131–135.

ICHIHARA, T., SUSUMI, S. and KURAMOTO, T. (1956) Studies on the diagnosis of fascioliasis. III. Precipitation test for fascioliasis in goats. *Jap. J. vet. Sci.,* **18**, 137–140.

ISODA, M., NAGANO, K., KIMINAMI, S. and AOYAGI, K. (1958) Studies on extermination of lymnaeid snails, intermediate host of *Fasciola hepatica* by raising carp in the paddy field. *J. Jap. vet. med. Ass.,* **11**, 72–74.

ITAGAKI, H. (1958) Relation between the prevalence of fascioliasis and the distribution of the snail intermediate host of the liver fluke. *Bull. Biograph. soc. Japan,* **20**, 29–32.

JAMIESON, S., THOMSON, J. J. and BROTHERTON, J. G. (1948) Studies in black disease. I. The occurrence of the disease in sheep in the north of Scotland. *Vet. Rec.,* **60**, 11–14.

JAMIESON, S. and THOMSON, A. (1949) Studies in black disease. II. The value of *Clostridium oedematiens* toxoid and anaculture together with carbon tetrachloride therapy in the control of the disease. *Vet. Rec.,* **61**, 299–402.

JAMIESON, S. (1949a) The identification of *Clostridium oedematiens* and an experimental investigation of its role in the pathogenesis of infectious necrotic hepatitis ("black disease" of sheep). *J. Path. Bact.,* **61**, 389–402.

JAMIESON, S. (1949b) Black disease of sheep. *Scot. Agric.,* **28**, 155–161.

JARRETT, W. H. F., JENNINGS, F. W., MARTIN, B., McINTYRE, W. I. M., MULLIGAN, W., SHARP, N. C. C. and URQUHART, G. M. (1958) A field trial of a parasitic bronchitis vaccine. *Vet. Rec.,* **70**, 451–454.

JEFFERIES, H. S. and DAWES, B. (Correspondence) (1960) Elucidation of the life cycle of *Fasciola hepatica*. *Nature,* **185,** 331–332.

JENNINGS, F. W., MULLIGAN, W. and URQUHART, G. M. (1955) Some isotopic studies on blood loss associated with *Fasciola hepatica* infection of rabbits. *Trans. R. Soc. trop. Med. Hyg.,* **49,** 305.

JENNINGS, F. W., MULLIGAN, W. and URQUHART, G. M. (1956) Radioisotope studies on the anemia produced by infection with *Fasciola hepatica*. *Exp. Parasit.,* **5,** 458–468.

JEPPS, M. W. (1933) Miracidia of the liver fluke for laboratory work. *Nature,* **132,** 171.

JOHN, B. (1953) The behaviour of the nucleus during the spermatogenesis in *Fasciola hepatica*. *Quart. J. micr. Sci.,* **94,** 41–55.

JOHNSTON, T. H. (1946) The transmitting agent of the sheep liver fluke in South Australia. *J. Dep. Agric. S. Aust.,* **50,** 194–197.

JOHNSTON, T. H. and BECKWITH, A. C. (1946) The life cycle of the sheep liver fluke in South Australia. *Trans. roy. Soc. S. Aust.,* **70,** 121–126.

JOHRI, L. N. and SMYTH, J. D. (1956) A histochemical approach to the study of helminth morphology. *Parasitology,* **46,** 107–116.

JOHRI, L. N. (1957) A morphological and histochemical study of egg formation in a cyclophyllidean Cestode. *Parasitology,* **47,** 21–29.

JORDAN, W. J. (1960) Treatment of fascioliasis. *Vet. Rec.,* **72,** 785.

JOSEPH, G. (1883) Vorläufige Mitteilung über die Jugendzustände der Leberegel. *Zool. Anz.,* **6,** 323.

JUDAH, J. D. and REES, K. R. (1959) Mechanism of action of CCl_4. (Symposium). *Fed. Proc.,* **18,** 1013–1016.

KAGRAMANOV, A. K. (1955) Experimental treatment of sheep with fascioliasis by subcutaneous application of carbon tetrachloride. *Veterinariya,* **32,** 39–40.

KAŠTÁK, V. (1958) Pastoinné vodojemy a ich funkcia v epizootologii fascolozy. *Veterinarsky Časopis, Bratislava,* **7,** 290–292.

KAWANA, H. (1940) Study on the development of the excretory system of *Fasciola hepatica* L. with special reference to its first intermediate host in Central China. *J. Shanghai Sci. Inst.,* **5,** 13–34.

KELLAWAY, C. H. (1928) Anaphylatic experiments with extracts of liver fluke (*Fasciola hepatica*). *Austr. Jour. exp. Biol. Med. Sci.,* **5,** 273–283.

KELLER, H. (1952) Zusammenhang der Lebertuberkulose mit Leberegelbefall. Dissertation, Munich, 1952.

KENDALL, S. B. (1949a) Species of Limnaea as intermediates hosts of *Fasciola hepatica*. *Vet. Rec.,* **61,** 462.

KENDALL, S. B. (1949b) *Lymnaea stagnalis* as an intermediate host of *Fasciola hepatica*. *Nature,* **163,** 880–881.

KENDALL, S. B. (1949c) Bionomics of *Limnaea truncatula* and the parthenitae of *Fasciola hepatica* under drought conditions. *J. Helminth,* **23,** 57–68.

KENDALL, S. B. (1949d) Nutritional factors affecting the rate of development of *Fasciola hepatica* in *Limnaea truncatula*. *J. Helminth,* **23,** 179–190.

KENDALL, S. B. (1950) Snail hosts of *Fasciola hepatica* in Britain. *J. Helminth.*, **24**, 63–74.

KENDALL, S. B. (1951) Carbon tetrachloride poisoning in cattle. *Vet. Rec.*, **63**, 716.

KENDALL, S. B. (1953) The life history of *Limnaea truncatula* under laboratory conditions. *J. Helminth.*, **27**, 17–28.

KENDALL, S. B. (1954) Fascioliasis in Pakistan. *Ann. trop. Med. Parasit.*, **48**, 307–313.

KENDALL, S. B. (1956) Liver flukes and snails in Asia. *Proc. Linn. Soc. Lond.*, **166**, 6.

KENDALL, S. B. and McCULLOUGH, F. S. (1951) The emergence of cercariae of *Fasciola hepatica* from the snail *Limnaea truncatula*. *J. Helminth.*, **25**, 77–92.

KENDALL, S. B. and PARFITT, J. W. (1953) Life history of *Fasciola gigantica* Cobbold 1856. *Nature (Lond.)*, **171**, 1164–1165.

KENDALL, S. B. and PARFITT, J. W. (1959) Studies on susceptibility of some species of *Lymnaea* to infection with *Fasciola gigantica* and *Fasciola hepatica*. *Ann. trop. Med. Parasit.*, **53**, 220–227.

KENDALL, S. B. and PARFITT, J. W. (1962) The chemotherapy of fascioliasis. *Brit. vet. J.*, **118**, 1–10.

KEOGH, J. (1955) Fascioliasis in South Australia. *Aust. vet. J.*, **31**, 48–49.

KERR, K. B. and PETKOVITCH, O. L. (1935) Active immunity in rabbits to the liver fluke, *Fasciola hepatica*. *J. Parasit.*, **21**, 319–320.

KHALIL, L. F. (1961) On the capture and destruction of miracidia by *Chaetogaster limnaei* (Oligochaeta). *J. Helminth.*, **35**, 269–274.

KHANBEGYAN, R. A (1956) Use of hexachlorethane in fascioliasis of cattle, sheep and goats. *Trud. armyansk. nauch.-issled. Inst. Zhivotn. veter.*, **9**, 101–106.

KIBAKIN, V. V. (1960) Epizootology of fascioliasis in sheep in the Tashauz region of the Turkmen S.S.R. *Trudi Turkmensk. Inst. Zhivotn. Veterin.*, **2**, 257–266.

KIBAKIN, V. V. (1961) The epizootology of fascioliasis in sheep in the Turkmen S.S.R. Conference (4th) on Problems in Parasitology, Alma Ata, 1959, 389–393.

KIMURA, S. (1961a) Experimental studies on Fascioliasis. I. Infection rate of metacercariae in rabbits, distribution of *Fasciola hepatica* in the liver, and the relation between the number of parasites and death of infected rabbits. *J. Parasit. Japan.*, **10**, 45–51.

KIMURA, S. (1961b) Experimental studies on Fascioliasis. II. Appearance of eggs in the faeces of infected rabbits. *J. Parasit. Japan*, **10**, 165–170.

KIMURA, S. (1961c) Experimental studies on fascioliasis. III. Clinical and haematological observations on infected rabbits. *J. Parasit. Japan*, **10**. 336–341.

KINGSCOTE, A. A. (1950) Liver rot (fascioloidiasis) in Ruminants. *Canad. J. Comp. Med.*, **14**, 203–208.

KLEKOVKIN, L. N. and SIPAKOV, V. N. (1958) An attempt to eradicate fascioliasis of domestic ruminants in the Magilev district. *Veterinariya,* **35,** 16–19.

KOCH, J. H. (1963) The toxic action of phenothiazine and some disturbances of intermediary metabolism in undernourished sheep. *Aust. J. agr. Res.,* **14,** 529–539.

KOCHNEV, P. N. (1950) *Fasciola* in the lungs of cattle. *Veterinariya,* **27,** 27.

KOKURICHEV, P. I. and KARBAINOV, M. A. (1957) Specificity of the tuberculin reaction in cattle infected with fascioliasis. *Sborn. Nauch. Trud.,* No. 11, 81–85.

KOMINE, S., USUI, M., WATANABE, S. and SUGIURA, M. (1955) Relationship between serum flocculation test and ratio of serum total proteins and fractions in bovine fascioliasis. *J. Jap. vet. med. Ass.,* **8,** 11–13.

KOMJÁTHY, K. (1957) Szarvasmarhák májmétylkóryának orvoslása lör alá fecskendezett széntetrakloriddal. *Magyar Allatorv. Lapja,* **12,** 235–236.

KOŇA, E. (1957a) Elektroforéza krvného śera oviec, chorýeh na fasciolózu. *Sborn. Ceskoslov. Akad. Vet. Med.,* **30,** 159–164.

KOŇA, E. (1957b) Elektroforeticke vysetrsovanie bielkovinovych frakeii krvneho sera a peritonealneho i perikardialneho exsudatu u oviec, choryeh na fasciolozu. *Veter. Casopis, Bratislava,* **6,** 146–150.

KOTLÁN, S. and KOVACS, F. (1957) Szarvasmarhak májmétyloyának gyógykezelése parenterálisan adott széntetetrakloriddal. *Magyar Allatorv. Lapja,* **12,** 65–66.

KOURI, P., BASNUEVO, J., ALVARÉ, L., LESCANO, O. and SIMON, R. (1931) Note previa sobre la genesis del huevo de *Fasciola hepatica. Rev.Parasit., Habana,* **2,** 173–174.

KOVACS, F. (1959) Die intramuskuläre Behandlung der Rinderfasziolose mit Tetrachlorkohlenstoff. *XVI Intern. Vet. Congress Madrid 1959,* **11,** 605–607.

KRUEDENER, R. VON (1952) Über die Ursachen der Aufwärtswanderung von *Bacterium coli* bei Rindern mit Leberegelbefall. Dissertation, Munich, 1952.

KRUDENIER, F. J. (1953) Studies on the encystation of larval digenetic trematodes. *J. Parasit.,* **39** (suppl.), 16.

KRULL, W. H. (1933) A new snail and rabbit host for *Fasciola hepatica* L. *J. Parasit.,* **20,** 49–52.

KRULL, W. H. (1933a) The snail *Pseudosuccinea columella* (Say) as a potentially important intermediate host in extending the range of *Fasciola hepatica* L. *J. Wash. Acad. Sci.,* **23,** 389–391.

KRULL, W. H. (1934) The intermediate hosts of *Fasciola hepatica* and *Fascioloides magna* in the United States. *N. Amer. Vet.,* **15,** 13–17.

KRULL, W. H. (1934b) Notes on the hatchability and infectivity of refrigerated eggs of *Fasciola hepatica* Linn. *Proc. Iowa Acad. Sci.,* **41,** 309.

KRULL, W. H. (1941) The number of cercariae of *Fasciola hepatica* developing in snails infected with a single miracidium. *Proc. helm. Soc. Wash.,* **8,** 55–58.

KRULL, W. H. and JACKSON, R. S. (1943) Observations on the route of migration of the common liver fluke, *Fasciola hepatica,* in the definitive host. *J. Wash. Acad. Sci.,* **33,** 79–82.

KÜMMEL, G. (1958) Das Terminalorgan der Protonephridien, Feinstruktur und Deutung der Funktion. *Z. Naturf.,* **13** B, 677–679.

KÜMMEL, G. (1960) Feinstruktur der Wimperflamme in der Protonephridien. *Protoplasma,* **51,** 371–376.

KURELEC, B., AUDI, S. and EHRLICH, I. (1961) Über die Verteilung des Atebrins bei *Fasciola hepatica. Exp. Parasit.,* **11,** 264–269.

KURELEC, B. and EHRLICH, I. (1963) Über die Natur der von *Fasciola hepatica* L. *in vitro* ausgeschiedenen amino- und ketosäuren. *Exper. Parasit.,* **13,** 113–117.

LAGRANGE, E. and SCHEECQMANS, G. (1950) Recherches expérimentales sur l'infestation à *Bilharzia mansoni* de la souris. *C. R. Soc. Belg. Biol.,* **144,** 1422–1424.

LAL, M. B. and SHRIVASTAVA, S. C. (1960) Some histochemical observations on the cuticle of *Fasciola indica* Varma 1953. *Experientia, Basle,* **16,** 185–186.

LÄMMLER, G. (1956) Die Chemotherapie der Fasciolose. II. Mitteilung über vergleichende experimentell-chemotherapeutische Untersuchungen an der Leberegelerkrankung des Kaninchens. *Z. Tropenmed. u. Parasit.,* **7,** 289–311.

LÄMMLER, G. (1959) Die Chemotherapie der Fasciolose. III. Mitteilung. Über die experimentelle *Fasciola hepatica* -Infektion der albino Ratte. *Tropenmed. u. Parasit.,* **10,** 379–384.

LÄMMLER, G. (1960) Chemotherapeutische Untersuchungen mit Hetol, einem neuen hochwirksamen Leberegelmittel. *Dtsch. tierärztl. Wschr.,* **67,** 408–413.

LÄMMLER, G. (1961) Die kombinierte Behandlung des Leberegels und Magendarmwürmerbefalls bei Schafen mit Hetol -R und Phenothiazins. *Dtsch. tierärztl. Wschr.,* **68,** 169–172.

LANG, A. (1880) Untersuchungen zur vergleichenden Anatomie und Histologie des Nervensystems der Plathelminthen. II. Über das Nervensystem der Trematoden. *Mitt. zool. Sta. Neapel,* **2,** 28–52.

LA RUE, G. R. (1957) The classification of digenetic Trematoda: A review and a new system. *Exp. Parasit.,* **6,** 306–349.

LAVIER, G. and STEFANOPOULO, G. (1944) L'intradermo-réaction et la réaction de fixation du complément dans la distomatose humaine à *Fasciola hepatica. Bull. Soc. Pat. exot.,* **37,** 302–308.

LEDERMAN, F. (1958) La distomatose bovine des régions du Sud-Kivu, Congo Belge. *Bull. Off. int. Epiz.,* **50,** 385–421.

LEIPER, J. W. G. (1938) The longevity of *Fasciola hepatica. J. Helminth.,* **16,** 173–176.

LEONTIEV, K. L. (1956) Diagnosis of *Fasciola hepatica* infection in live cattle. *Veterinariya,* **33,** 46.

LEUCKART, R. (1881) Zur Entwicklungsgeschichte des Leberegels. *Zool. Anz.*, **99**, 641–646.

LEUCKART, R. (1882a) Zur Entwicklungsgeschichte des Leberegels (*Distomum hepaticum*). *Arch. Naturgesch.*, **48**, 80–119.

LEUCKART, R. (1882b) Zur Entwicklungsgeschichte des Leberegels. Zweite Mittheilung. *Zool. Anz.*, **122**, 524–528.

LIENERT, E. (1949) Kymographische Versuche über die Wirkung organischer Farbstoffe auf den grossen Leberegel (*Fasciola hepatica*). *Wien Tierärztl. Mschr.*, **36**, 650–659.

LIENERT, E. and MATHOIS, H. (1952a) Prüfung weiterer mit der Galle ausscheidbarer Arzneimittel auf Leberegelwirksamkeit. *Wien. Tierärztl. Mschr.*, **39**, 344–352.

LIENERT, E. and MATHOIS, H. (1952b) Untersuchungen zur Ermittlung noch stärker leberegelwirksamer Substanzen. *Wien. Tierärztl. Mschr.*, **39**, 410–146.

LIENERT, E. (1959) Experimentelle Untersuchungen zur Chemotherapie der Distomatose. II. Mitteilung. Implantation geschlechtsreifer Exemplare von *Fasciola hepatica* L. unter die Rückenhaut der weissen Ratte. *Wien. Tierärztl. Mschr.*, **46**, 423–430.

LIENERT, E. (1960) Die Wirkung von Aureomycin auf unter die Rückenhaut der weissen Ratte implantierte geschlechtsreife Exemplare von *Fasciola hepatica* L. *Wien. Tierärztl. Mschr.*, **47**, 313–318.

LIENERT, E. (1960b) Die durch Hexachlorophen erzielbare tödliche Wirkung auf den grossen Leberegel (*Fasciola hepatica* L.) wird durch das Blut des Wirtes vermittelt. *Chemotherapie*, **1**, 384–391.

LIENERT, E. (1960c) Erläuterungen zum "Leberegeltest". *Wien. Tierärztl. Mschr.*, **47**, 677–683.

LIENERT, E. (1961) Leberegeltest. *Exp. Parasit.*, **10**, 223–225.

LIENERT, E. (1962) Bithionol (Actamer) ist im "Leberegeltest" Fasciola hepatica wirksam. *Z. Tropenmed. Paras.*, **13**, 338–341.

LIENERT, E. and JAHN, F. (1962a) Prüfung von Bromchlorophen im Leberegeltest. *Wien. Tierärztl. Mschr.*, **49**, 829–832.

LIENERT, E. and JAHN, F. (1962b) Prüfung von Halothan (Fluothane im) "Leberegeltest". *Wien. Tierärztl. Mschr.*, **49**, 928–932.

LIENERT, E. (1963a) A positive result can be transferred from the "liver fluke test" to cattle infested with *Fasciola hepatica* L. *Wien. Tierärztl. Mschr.*, **50**, 217–221.

LIENERT, E. (1963b) Diaphene ist im "Leberegeltest" *Fasciola hepatica* wirksam. *Arch. exp. vet. Med.*, **16**, 101–104.

LOGACHEV, E. D. (1960) On the trophic function of the intestinal epithelium of Trematodes. *Dokl. Ac. Sci. U.R.S.S.* (Translation), **131**, 282–284.

LOGACHEV, E. D. (1961) On the structure and development of supporting structures of internal tissue of Trematodes. *Dokl. Ac. Sci. U.R.S.S.* (Translation), **133**, 599–601.

Looss, A. (1885) Beiträge zur Kenntnis der Trematoden. *Z. wiss. Zool.*, **41,** 390–446.

Lunedei, A. and Rosselli del Turco, L. (1934) Il primo caso nell' uomo di metastais cerebrale di *Fasciola hepatica* in soggetto osservato in Italia. Considerazioni generali sulla distomatosi umana da fasciola. *Rev. Clin. Medica,* **35,** 465–498.

Lungu, V., Georgescu, L., Fromunda, V. and Stoican, E. (1959) Cercetări privind asanarea pasunilov contaminate fascioloza. *Lucrarile Stiintifice ale Institutului de Patologie si Igiena Animalia, Bucharest,* **9,** 315–323.

Lungu, V., Stoican, E., Fromunda, V. and Drafusin, A. (1960) Tratamentul fasciolozei ovine cu amestec uleios de tetrachlorura de carbon si hexacloretan prin administrare parenterala. *Lucrarile Stiintifice ale Institului de Patologie si Igiena Animalia, Bucharest,* **9,** 315–323.

Lungu, V. (1959) Die Leberegelseuche in der Rumänischen Volksrepublik (Epizootologie und Bekämpfung). *Wiad. Parazyt.,* **5,** 345–355.

Ma, L. (1963) Trace elements and plyphenol oxidase in *Clonorchis sinensis. J. Paras.,* **49,** 197–203.

McCauley, J. E. (1958) A new method for examining snails for Trematode parasites. *J. Parasitol.,* **44,** 243.

McGraw, B. M. (1959) The ecology of the snail *Lymnaea humilis. Trans. Amer. micr. Soc.,* **78,** 101–121.

Macé, E. (1881) Recherches anatomiques sur la grande douve du foie. Thèse de médecine, Paris

Mackie, A., Stewart, G. H. and Misra, A. L. (1955) *In vitro* testing of benzoltriazols and some phenothiazine derivatives against lumbricoids of *Fasciola hepatica. Arch. int. Pharmacodyn.,* **103,** 187–191.

Maekawa, K., Kitazawa, K. and Kushibe, M. (1954) Purification et cristallisation de l'antigène pour la dermo-réaction allergique vis-à-vis de *Fasciola hepatica. C. R. Soc. Biol., Paris,* **148,** 763–765.

Maekawa, K. and Kushibe, M. (1956) Sur la composition chimique de l'antigène pour la dermo-réaction allergique viv-à-vis de *Fasciola hepatica. C. R. Soc. Biol. Paris,* **150,** 832–834.

Maglaulić, E., Ožegović, L. and Turančić, V. (1959) Labilitetni pokusi serumkih bjelančevina i protrombinsko vrijeme kod distomatoze goveda. *Veterinaria Sarajevo,* **8,** 229–233.

Manokyan, Z. K. (1955) Non-specific tuberculin reaction in cattle with fascioliasis. *Trudi Armyansk. Navchno-Issl. Vet. Inst.,* **8,** 25–28.

Mansour, T. E. (1957a) The effect of lysergic acid, diethylamide 5-hydroxytryptamine and related compounds on liver fluke, *Fasciola hepatica. Brit. J. Pharmacol.,* **12,** 406–409.

Mansour, T. E. (1957b) Studies on the phenol oxidase of *Fasciola hepatica. Amer. J. trop. Med. Hyg.,* **6,** 391–392.

Mansour, T. E. (1958) Effect of serotonin on phenol oxidase from the liver fluke *Fasciola hepatica* and from other sources. *Biochim. biophys. Acta,* **30,** 492–500.

Mansour, T. E. (1959) Action of serotonin and epinephrine on intact and broken cell preparations of the liver fluke. *Pharmacol. Rev.,* **11,** 465–466.

MANSOUR, T. E., SUTHERLAND, E. W., RALL, T. W. and BUEDING, E. (1960) The effect of serotonin (5-hydroxytryptamine) on the formation of adenosine 3′,5′-phosphate by tissue particles from the liver fluke, *Fasciola hepatica. J. biol. Chem.*, **235**, 466–470.

MANSOUR, T. E. (1962) Effects of serotonin on glycolysis in homogenates from the liver fluke *Fasciola hepatica. J. Pharm. exp. Ther.*, **135**, 94-101.

MANSOUR, T. E. and MANSOUR, J. M. (1962) Effects of serotonin (5-hydroxytryptamine) and adenosine 3′,5′-phosphate on phosphofructokinase from the liver fluke, *Fasciola hepatica. J. biol. Chem.*, **237**, 629–634.

MARCHEBOEUF, M. and MANDOUL, R. (1939a) A propos de la toxicité des extraits d'*Ascaris. C. R. Soc. Biol. Paris*, **130**, 1032–1034.

MARCHEBOEUF, M. and MANDOUL, R. (1939b) Tentative d'isolement de la substance toxique contenue dans l'extrait d'*Ascaris megalocephala.* Quelques observations au sujet des propriétés de cette substance. *C. R. Soc. Biol. Paris,* **132**, 124–126.

MAREK, J. (1927) Neuere Beiträge zur Kenntnis der Leberegelkrankheit mit besonderer Berücksichtigung der Infektionweise, der Entwicklung der Distomum, und der Therapie. *Dtsch. tierärztl. Wschr.,* **34**, 513–519.

MARTINEZ DE JESUS, J. and RIVERA-ANAYA, J. D. (1952) An improved technique for the microscopic diagnosis of liver fluke infection in cattle. *J. Amer. vet. med. Ass.,* **120**, 203–204.

MARZULLO, F., SQUADRINI, F. and TADARELLI, F. (1957) Studio istochimico sui parasiti patogeni per l'uomo. III. Uova dei *F. hepatica* e *Dicrocoelium dendriticum. Boll. Soc. med.-chir. Modena,* **57**, 501–505.

MASU, S. (1955) Studies on protein and polysaccharide antigens of *Fasciola hepatica. Sci. Rep. Ayuba Vet. Coll., Japan,* No. 2, 69–78.

MATTÉS, O. (1926) Zur Biologie der Larvenentwicklung von *Fasciola hepatica,* besonders über den Einfluss der Wasserstoffionkonzentration auf das Ausschlüpfen der Miracidien. *Zool. Anzeiger,* **69**, 138–156.

MATTÉS, O. (1949) Wirtsfindung, Invasionsvorgang und Wirtsspezifität beim *Fasciola* miracidium. *Z. Parasitenk.,* **14**, 320–363.

MAYER, M. and PIFANO, C. F. (1945) La especifidad de las intradermoreacciones eomparativas con extracto de *Schistosoma mansoni* y *Fasciola hepatica* en el diagnostico de la Bilharziosis. *Rev. Sanid. y Asist. Soc., Caracas,* **10**, 45–49.

MAZOTTI, L. (1948) Aplicación de la intradermorreacción en casos humanos de infección por *Fasciola hepatica. Rev. Inst. Salubr. Enferm. trop., Méx.,* **9**, 257–261.

MAZOTTI, L. (1955) *Lymnaea obrussa Say,* huesped intermediario de *Fasciola hepatica. Rev. Inst. Sal. Enferm. Trop., Mexico,* **15**, 163–165.

MCCAULEY, J. E. (1958) A new method for examining snails for Trematode parasites. *J. Parasitol.,* **44**, 243.

MCGRAW, B. M. (1959) The ecology of the snail *Lymnaea humilis. Trans. amer. micr. Soc.,* **78**, 101–121.

MEHL, S. (1932) Die Lebensbedingungen der Leberegelschnecke (*Galba truncatula* Muller). *Arb. bayer. Landesanst. Pfl. Bau.* No. 10, Freising, München 1933.

MEHLIS, C. F. E. (1831) *Novae observationes de Entozois*. Isis von Oken, Jahrg. 1831, 68–99 and 166–199.

MERLEN, H. (1950) *Fasciola hepatica* and the tuberculin reaction. *Vet. Rec.,* **62**, 570.

METTRICK, D. F. and TELFORD, J. M. (1963) Histamine in the phylum Platyhelminthes. *J. Parasit.,* **49**, 653–656.

MICHELSON, E. H. (1957) Predators and parasites of fresh water mollusca: a review of the literature. *Parasitology,* **47**, 413–426.

MICHAESCU, N., STOICAN, E. and SUTEU, E. (1953) Diagnositicul alergic in ascaridioza pereina se distomatoza ovina. *Anuarul Institutului de Patologie Igiena Animala, Bucharest,* **4**, 266–272.

MIKACIC, D. (1959) Odnos izmedu koproloskog nalaza i stupnja invazije velikim metiljem (*Fasciola hepatica*) u goveda. *Vet. Arhiv.,* **29**, 244–249.

MINNING, W. and FUHRMANN, C. (1955) Protein- Kohlehydrat- und Lipoid-Fracktionen von *Fasciola hepatica* als KBR-Antigene. *Z. Tropenmed. u. Parasit.,* **6**, 92–99.

MINNING, W., NEWSOME, J. and ROBINSON, D. L. H. (1958) Trematoden-Stoffwechselprodukte als Antigene. *Z. Tropenmed. u. Parasit.,* **9**, 335–342.

MINNING, W., and VOGEL, H. (1950) Immunobiologische und epidemiologische Untersuchungen bei drei Fällen von menschlicher Fasciolose. *Z. Tropenmed. u. Parasit.,* **1**, 532–553.

MITTERPAK, J. (1958) Profylakticka dehelmintizacia, zaklad boja s fasciolozou domacich zvierat. *Sbornik Ceskoslovenske Akademie Zemedelskych ved Veterinarni Medicina,* **31**, 981–992.

MONNÉ, L. (1959) On the external cuticles of various helminths and their role in the host-parasite relationship. *Ark. Zool.,* **12**, 343–358.

MONNET, P., COUDERT, J., CORNUT, P. and BRETTE, R. (1950) Distomatose a symptomatologie anormale ou compliquee de greffe infectieuse sur une cardiopathie ancienne? Valeur de l'intradermo-reaction a l'antigene de douve. Echec du glucantine. Guerison de l'etat septisemique par la chloromycetine. *Lyon Med.,* **183**, 427–431.

MONNET, P., COUDERT, J., CORNUT, P. and BRETTE, R. (1951) Précocité de l'intra-dermo-réaction à l'extrait de douve. Valeur diagnostique dans un cas de distomatose à symptomatologie anormale et compliqué. *J. Med., Bordeaux,* **128**, 252–253.

MONTGOMERIE, R. F. (1928) Observations on artificial infestation of sheep with *Fasciola hepatica* and on a phase in the development of the parasite. *J. Helminth,* **6**, 167–174.

MONTGOMERIE, R. F. (1931) On the longevity of *Fasciola hepatica* in experimentally infected rabbits. *J. Helminth.,* **9**, 209–212.

MORENAS, L. (1944) Le diagnostic biologique de la distomatose hepatique: essai de cuti et d'intradermoreactions. *Lyon Medical,* **171**, 51–66.

MORRIL, D. R. and Shaw, J. N. (1942) Studies of the pathology in cattle produced by liver fluke. *Ore. Agri. exp. Sta. Bull.,* No. 408.

MOZLEY, A. (1957) *Liver fluke snails in Britain.* Lewis & Co.

MUCHLIS, A. (1959) Distomatosis paru pada biri. *Hemera zoa,* **66**, 71–74.

MÜLLER, W. (1923) Die Nahrung von *Fasciola hepatica* und ihre Verdauung. *Zool. Anz.,* **57,** 273–281.

MÜLLER, O. F. (1773–1774) Vermium terrestrium et fluviatilium . . . succincta historia. *Hafniae et Lipsiae,* vol. I (1): Infusoria.

MUNOZ-RIVAS, G. (1954) Fascioliasis experimental. *Rev. Acad. Colomb.,* **9,** 156–158.

MURAVEV, L. D. (1950) Atypical fascioliasis in sheep. *Veterinariya,* **27,** 28–29.

NEUHAUS, W. (1936) Der Invasionsweg der Lanzettegelcercariae bei der Infektion des Endwirtes und ihre Entwicklung zum *Dicrocoelium lanceatum. Z. Parasitenk.,* **10,** 476–512.

NEUHAUS, W. (1953) Über den chemischen Sinn der Miracidien von *Fasciola hepatica. Z. Parasitenk,* **15,** 476–490.

NOGUCHI, I., KIRISAWA, T., SUGIURA, K. and KOMINE, S. (1958) Studies on liver function tests. 1. Liver function tests on sheep infected with liver fluke. *J. Jap. vet. med. Ass.,* **11,** 113–115.

ÖKLAND, F. (1934) Utlredelse og hyppighet an den store leverikte (*Fasciola hepatica* L.) i Norge. *Norsk. Vet. Tidsskr.,* 7–9.

ÖKLAND, F. (1935) *Limnaea truncatula* regulating the occurrence of *Fasciola hepatica* in Norway. *Zoogeographia,* **3,** 16–26.

OLIVER GONZALEZ, J., RIVERA ANAYA, J. D. and MARTINEZ DE JESUS (1950) Intradermal reactions in cattle to antigen prepared from *Fasciola hepatica. Puerto Rico J. publ. Hlth. trop. Med.,* **26,** 121–124.

OLLERENSHAW, C. B. (1958a) Climate and liver fluke disease in Anglesey. *Trans. R. Soc. trop. Med. Hyg.,* **52,** 303.

OLLERENSHAW, C. B. (1958b) Climate and liver flukes. *Agriculture, Lond.,* **65,** 231–235.

OLLERENSHAW, C. B. (1959) Ecology of liver fluke (*Fasciola hepatica*). *Vet. Rec.,* **71,** 957–963.

OLLERENSHAW, C. B. (1962) The control of fascioliasis — the need for a planned approach. *Outlook in Agric.,* **3,** 278–281.

OLLERENSHAW, C. B. and ROWLANDS, W. T. (1959) A method of forecasting the incidence of fascioliasis in Anglesey. *Vet. Rec.,* **71,** 591–598.

OLSEN, O. W. (1944) Bionomics of the lymnaeid snail, *Stagnicola bulimoides techella,* the intermediate host of the liver fluke in southern Texas. *J. agric. Res.,* **69,** 389–493.

OLSEN, O. W. (1945) Ecology of the metacercariae of *Fasciola hepatica* in southern Texas and its relationship to liver fluke control in cattle. *J. Parasit.,* **31** (suppl.) 20.

OLSEN, O. W. (1947) Hexachlorethane-bentonite suspension for controlling the common liver fluke *Fasciola hepatica* in cattle in the gulf coast region of Texas. *Amer. J. vet. Res.,* **8,** 353–366.

OLSEN, O. W. (1948) Wild rabbits as reservoir hosts of the common liver fluke *Fasciola hepatica* in southern Texas. *J. Parasit.,* **34,** 119–123.

OLSEN, O. W. (1949) Liver fluke in cattle: Diagnosis for treatment and prevention. *Proc. U.S. live Stk. sanit. Assoc.* (1948 Meeting), 79–93.

ONO, Y., *et al.* (1957) Studies on *Limnaea pervia* as an intermediate host of *Fasciola hepatica* in Hyogo Perfecture. *J. Jap. vet. med. Ass.,* **10**, 227–230.

ONO, Y. (1958) Infestation des Ruminants par la douve. *Bull. Off. Intern. Epiz.,* **49**, 550–554.

ONO, Y. and ISODA, M. (1951) Studies on the fascioliasis. I. Observations on the life-history of *Fasciola hepatica. Jap. J. vet. Sci.,* **13**, 87–96.

ONO, M. and WATANABE, S. (1956) Studies on the polysaccharides in the antigen of skin test for bovine fascioliasis. *Jap. J. Vet. Sc.,* **18**, 141–148.

ONO, M., WATANABE, S. and AKUZEWA, M. (1956) Studies on freeze dried antigen for intradermal reaction of *Fasciola hepatica. J. Japan. Vet. Med. Ass.,* **9**, 415–417.

ORTMANN, W. (1908) Zur Embryonalentwicklung des Leberegels (*Fasciola hepatica*). *Zool. Jb.,* **26**, 255–292.

ORTNER-SCHÖNBACH, P. (1913) Zur Morphologie des Glykogens bei Trematoden und Cestoden. *Arch. Zellforsch.,* **11**, 413–449.

OSHANOVA, N. (1959) Hibernation of parthenogenetic forms of Fasciola hepatica L. in the Sofia region. *Wiad. Parazyt.,* **5**, 357–359.

PACCANARO, A. (1909) La deviazione del complemento nelle distomiasi. *La Clin. Vet.,* No. 1.

PANASYUK, D. I. (1953) *The effect of hexachlorethane on the organism of the horse.* Izdatelstvo, Akademii Nauk. S.S.S.R. (Moscow), 470–482.

PANOVA, L. G. (1953) An experiment on the introduction of a complex method of control of fascioliasis in sheep into the practice of collective farms in the Tikhuin district of the Leningrad region. *Izdatelstvo Akademii Nauk. S.S.S.R. (Moscow),* 483–487.

PANTELOURIS, E. M. and GRESSON, R. A. R. (1960) Autoradiographic studies on *Fasciola hepatica* L. *Parasitology,* **50**, 165–169.

PANTELOURIS, E. M. and HALE, P. A. (1962) Iron and Vitamin C in *Fasciola hepatica* L. *Res. Vet. Sci.,* **3**, 300–303.

PANTELOURIS, E. M. and THREADGOLD, L. T. (1963) The excretory system of the adult *Fasciola hepatica* L. *La Cellule.*

PANTELOURIS, E. M. (1964a) Sulfur uptake by *Fasciola hepatica* L. *Life Sciences,* **3**, 1–5.

PANTELOURIS, E. M. (1964b) Localisation of glycogen in *Fasciola hepatica L.* and an effect of insulin. *J. Helminth,* **38**, 283–286.

PANTELOURIS, E. M. (1964c) Utilisation of methionine by the liver fluke, *Fasciola hepatica.* (In press).

PANTELOURIS, E. M. (1964d) Effects of host hormones on the internal parasite, *Fasciola hepatica.* (In press).

PARKER, W. H. (1948) Black disease in Shropshire and the prophylactic effect of *Clostridium oedematiens* serum. *Vet. Rec.,* **60**, 417.

PARNELL, I. W., RAYSKI, C., DUNN, A. M. and MACKINTOSH, G. M. (1954) A survey of the helminths of Scottish hill sheep. *J. Helminth.,* **28**, 53–100.

PARRY, J. A. (1959) Intramuscular carbon tetrachloride treatment of acute fascioliasis in sheep. *Vet. Rec.,* **71**, 536–537.

PATNAIK, B. and DAS K. M. (1961) Diagnosis of Fascioliasis in cattle by intradermal allergic test. *Cornell Vet.,* **51,** 113–123.

PAUTRIZEL, R., BAILANGER, J., DURET, J. and TRIBOULEY, J. (1962) Etude de la specificité d'un extrait antigenique de *Fasciola hepatica* dans les tests d'allergie cutanée. *Ann. Inst. Pasteur,* **103,** 778–785.

PAUTRIZEL, R. BEZIAU, A. and BAILANGER, J. (1949) Etudes sur la toxicité des helminths. I. Leur teneur en histamine. *Ann. Parasit. hum. comp.,* **24,** 460–463.

PAUTRIZEL, R., RIVASSEAU, J. and RIVASSEAU, D. (1951) Injection d'extrait de douve et éosinophilie sanguine chez le mouton douvé. *C. R. Soc. Biol.,* **145,** 720–721.

PEARSON, I. G. and BORAY, J. C. (1961) The anthelmintic effect of intramuscular injection of carbon tetrachloride on *Fasciola hepatica* in cattle. *Aust. Vet. J.,* **37,** 73–78.

PEARSON, L. G. (1963) Use of chromium radioisotope Cr-51 to estimate blood loss through ingestion by *Fasciola hepatica. Exp. Parasit.,* **13,** 186–193.

PECK, E. F. (1957) An operational knackery survey in Devon, 1953–6. *Vet. Rec.,* **69,** 939–946.

PENNOIT-DE COOMAN, E. and VAN GREMBERGEN, G. (1942) Vergelijkend onderzoek van het fermentensysteem bij vrijlevende en parasitaire Plathelminthen. *Verhand. Koninkl. Vlaamsche Ahad., Wetensch.,* **4,** No. 6 (pp.1–77).

PENSO, G. and VIANELLO, G. (1937) La calcionamide nella lotta contro le distomatosi. *Clin. Vet.,* **60,** 711–715.

PETERS, B. G. and CLAPHAM, P. A. (1942) Infestation with liver fluke among 73000 cattle slaughtered in Great Britain during June, 1942. *J. Helminth.,* **20,** 115–138.

PETERS, B. G. (1938) Habitats of *Limnaea truncatula* in England and Wales during dry seasons. *J. Helminth.,* **16,** 213–260.

PETROCHENKO, V. I. (1954) The role of *Galba truncatula* in the distribution of fascioliasis. *Zoologicheski Zhurnal,* **33,** 44–49.

PRICE, E. W. (1953) The fluke situation in American ruminants. *J. Parasitol.,* **39,** 119–134.

POIRIER, M. and DESCHIENS, R. (1961) Etude histo-pathologique comparée des glandes surrénales dans les hyperéosinophilies parasitaires et non parasitaires. *Bull. Soc. Pat. exot.,* **54,** 212–215.

POLISHCHUK, F. G. and CHUPRINOVA, A. S. (1955) Fascioliasis in nutria. *Veterinariya,* **32,** 44.

POTEMKINA, V. A. (1945) Treatment of Fasciola in cattle with hexachlorethane. *Veterinariya,* **22,** 28–29.

PRENANT, M. (1922) Rechereches sur le parenchyme des Plathelminthes. *Arch. Morph. gén. exp.,* No. 5.

PRENANT, M. (1938) Quelques remarques sur le tégument des Trématodes digénétiques. *Bull. Soc. zool. Franc.,* **53,** 18–29.

PURCHASE, H. S. (1957) How important is liver fluke disease in South Africa? *J. S. Afr. vet. med. Ass.,* **28,** 337–340.

QUERNER, F. R. (1929) Zur Histologie des Exkretionssystems digenetischer Trematoden. *Zschr. Parasitenk.*, **1**, 489–561.

RAILLIET, A., MOUSSU, G. and HENRY, A. (1913) Recherches expérimentales sur le développement de la douve hépatique (*Fasciola hepatica* L.). *Rec. Med. vét.*, **90**, 1–6.

RAMIREZ VILLAMEDIANA, J. J. and VERGANI, F. (1949) Contribucion al estudio del ciclo evolutivo de la *Fasciola hepatica* en Venezuela. *Rev. grancolomb. Zootec.*, **3**, 817–38.

RANZOLI, F. (1955) Osservazioni preliminari sulle cellule vitelline e gli ovociti di *Fasciola hepatica* L. *R. c. Accad. Lincei*, **19**, 171–177.

RANZOLI, F. (1956) Cellule vitelline e ovociti in *Fasciola hepatica*. *Boll. Zool.*, **23**, 557–564.

RAO, K. H. (1959a) Observations on the Mehlis' gland complex in the liver fluke, *Fasciola hepatica*. *J. Parasit.* **45**, 347–351.

RAO, K. H. (1959b) Histochemistry of Mehlis' gland and egg-shell formation in the liver fluke. *Experientia*, **15**, 464.

RAO, K. H. (1960) The problem of Mehli's gland. *Parasitology*, **50**, 349–350.

REES, F. G. (1932) An investigation into the occurrence, structure and life histories of the trematode parasites of four species of *Lymnaea* (*truncatula, pereger, palustris, stagnalis*). *Proc. zool. Soc. Lond.*, **1**, 1–32.

REES, K. R., SINHA, K. P. and SPECTOR, W. G. (1961) The pathogenesis of liver injury in CCl_4 and thioacetamide poisoning. *J. Path. Bact.*, **81**.

REFUERZO, P. G. (1947) The treatment of fascioliasis in dairy cattle and in Indian buffaloes with hexachlorethane and kamala extract. *Philipp. J. Sci.*, **77**, 25–37.

REINHARD, E. G. (1957) Landmarks of parasitology. I. Discovery of the life cycle of liver fluke. *Exp. Parasit.*, **6**, 208–232.

RIDLEY, D. S. and HAWGOOD, B. C. (1956) The value of formol-ether concentration of faecal cysts and ova. *J. clin. Path.*, **9**, 74–76.

RIJAVEC, M., KURELEC, B. and EHRLICH, I. (1962) Über den Verbrauch der Serumalbumine *in vitro* durch *Fasciola hepatica*. *Biol. Glasnik*, **15**, 103–107.

RIVERA-ANAYA, J. D. and MARTINEZ DE JESUS, J. (1952) The extent of liver fluke infestation of cattle in Puerto Rico. (A slaughter house survey). *Bull. Puerto Rico agri. exp. Sta.*, No. 107, 16.

RIVERA-ANAYA, J. D., CIORDA, H. and MARTINEZ DE JESUS, J. (1953) Comparative efficiency of intradermal and precipitin tests in the diagnosis of fascioliasis of cattle in Puerto Rico. *Bull. P. R.* (*ins.*) *agric. Exp. Sta.*, No. 115, 20 pp.

ROBERTS, E. W. (1950) Studies on the life cycle of *Fasciola hepatica* (Linnaeus) and of its snail host, *Limnaea* (*Galba*) *truncatula* (Muller) in the field and under controlled conditions in the laboratory. *Ann. trop. Med. Parasit.*, **44**, 187–206.

ROBERTS, E. J. (1959) Problems of welsh agriculture. *Agriculture, Lond.*, **66**, 166–170.

Q

ROHRBACHER, G. H. (Jr.) (1957) Observations on the survival *in vitro* of bacteria-free adult common liver fluke, *Fasciola hepatica* Linn. 1758. *J. Parasit.*, **43**, 9–18.

ROLLESTON, G. (1880a) On the rot in sheep. *Zool. Anz.*, **3**, 258–260.

ROLLESTON, G. (1880b) Note on the geographical distribution of *Limax agrestis, Arion hortensis* and *Fasciola hepatica. Zool. Anz.*, **3**, 400–405.

ROMANINI, M. G. (1947) Contributo alla conoscenza istochimica dei vitellogeni di Distomum hepaticum. *Mon. zool. ital.*, **56**, 3–6.

ROSS, I. C. (1930) Some observations on the bionomics of *Fasciola hepatica. Jap. J. exp. Med.*, **8**, 65–69.

ROSS, I. C. and McKAY, A. C. (1929) The development of *Fasciola hepatica* L. in the final host. *Aust. Vet. J.*, **5**, 17–23.

ROSS, K. and McKAY, A. C. (1929) The bionomics of *Fasciola hepatica* in New South Wales and of the intermediate host *Limnaea brazieri. Bull. Coun. sci. industr. Res. Aust.*, **43**, 1–62.

ROTHMAN, A. (1958) The role of the bile salts in the biology of tapeworms. *Exp. Parasit.*, **7**, 328–337.

ROTHMAN, A. (1959) The role of bile salts in the biology of the tapeworms. II. Further observations on the effects of bile salts on metabolism. *J. Parasit.*, **45**, 379–383.

ROWAN, W. B. (1956) Mode of hatching of the egg of *Fasciola hepatica. Exp. Parasit.*, **5**, 118–137.

ROWCLIFFE, S. A. and OLLERENSHAW, C. B. (1960) Observations on the bionomics of the egg of *Fasciola hepatica. Ann. trop. Med. Parasit.*, **54**, 172–181.

RUKAWINA, W. (1935) *Leberegelerkrankung beim Menschen.* Lejecnicki Vjesnik, p. 326.

SAITO, A. (1961) Histochemical study on the digestive tract of *Fasciola hepatica. J. Tokyo Med. Coll.*, **19**, 1487–1497.

SALLNÄS, T. (1954) Svara angrepp av leveflundra i Östsverige, *Lantmannen*, **38**, 1130–1133.

SALUTINI, E. (1959) Il comportamento della chetonemia in bovine affette de parassitosi epatiche. *Ann. Fac. Med. Vet., Pisa*, **11**, 209–218.

SANDERSON, A. R. (1953) Maturation and probable gynogenesis in the liver fluke *Fasciola hepatica* L. *Nature*, **172**, 110–112.

SANDERSON, A. R. (1959) Maturation and fertilisation in two digentic trematodes, *Haplometra cylindracea* (Zeder 1800) and *Fasciola hepatica* (L.). *Proc. Soc. exp. Biol.*, **96**, 204–210.

SARWAR, M. M. (1957) *Fasciola indica* Varma, a synonym of *F. gigantica* Cobbold. *Biologia, Lahore*, **3**, 168–175.

SARWAR, M. M. and BARYA, M. A. (1960) Some observations on the use of carbon tetrachloride in fascioliasis in the field. *Proc. Pakistan Sci. Confer.* (12th), 12–13.

SAZANOV, A. M. (1957) Epizootiology and control of fascioliasis in ruminants. *Veterinariya*, **34**, 28–30.

SCHADIN, W. I. (1937) Einige Feld- und experimentelle Untersuchungen an *L. truncatula* Müll., dem Überträger der Fasciolosis. *Trans. Inst. Zool. Acad. Sci. USSR,* **4,** 541–564.

SCHAPER, A. (1889) Die Leberegelkrankheit der Haussäugethiere. Eine ätiologische und pathologisch-anatomische Untersuchung. *Dtsch. Z. Thiermed. vergl. Pathol.,* **16,** 1–95.

SCHINDLER, S. (1951) Über die Coli-agglutininbildung im Blutserum von Haustieren mit besonderer Berücksichtigung leberegelkranker Schafe. Dissertation, Münich, 1951.

SCHMID, F. (1934) Die Verbreitung des Leberegels in Bayern. *Z. Parasitenk.,* **6,** 528–545.

SCHMIDT-HOENSDORF, F. (1959) Ecobol, ein subcutan-verabreichbares Leberegelmittel. *Wiad. Parazyt.,* **5,** 335–339.

SCHUBMANN, W. (1905) Über die Eibildung und Embryonalentwicklung von *Fasciola hepatica* L. *Zool. Jb. Anat.,* **21,** 571–606.

SCHUMACHER, W. (1938) Untersuchungen über den Wanderweg und Entwicklung von *Fasciola hepatica* L. im Endwirt. *Z. Parasitenk.,* **10,** 608–643.

SCHUMACHER, W. (1956) Untersuchungen über das Eindringen der Jugendformen von *Fasciola hepatica* L. in der Leber des Endwirts. *Z. Parasitenk.,* **17,** 276–281.

SCHWARTZ, B., 1947. *Drugs to control parasites.* Yearb. U.S., Dep. Agric. (1947), 71–80.

SCHWARZ, K. (1960) Factor 3, selenium and vitamin E. *Nutr. Rev.,* **18,** 193–197.

SEKARDI, L. and EHRLICH, I. (1962) Acetilkolinesteraza velikog metilja (*Fasciola hepatica* L.) *Biol. Glasnik.,* **15,** 229–233.

SEMICHON, L. (1933) Sur le contenu des cellules vésiculeuses du parenchyme de *Fasciola hepatica* L. *C. R. Acad. Polon. Sci. Lettres,* **114,** 1179–1180.

SERVANTIE, L. (1921) Recherche de la déviation du complément dans la distomatose humaine. *C. R. Soc. Biol.,* **134,** 699.

SHAGINYAN, E. G. (1955) Mass treatment of fascioliasis in buffaloes with carbon tetrachloride. *Trud. armyansk. nauch.-issled. veter. Inst.,* **8,** 143–149.

SHARAF, A., HAIBA, M. H. and SHIHATA, I. M. (1960) *In vitro* studies on the effect of some anti-malarial drugs on *Fasciola* worms in buffaloes, cattle and sheep. *Amer. J. vet. Res.,* **21,** 308–310.

SHAW, J. N. and SIMMS, B. T. (1929) *Galba bulimoides Lea* as intermediate host of *Fasciola hepatica* in Oregon. *Science,* **69,** 357.

SHAW, J. N. (1931) Some notes on liver fluke investigations. *J. Amer. vet. med. Ass.,* **31,** 19–24.

SHAW, J. N. (1932) Studies of the liver fluke (*Fasciola hepatica*). *J. Amer. vet. med. Ass.,* **81,** 76–82.

SHAW, J. N. (1946) Further trials with hexachloroethane as a treatment for liver fluke in Oregon cattle. *N. Amer. Vet.,* **27,** 625–627.

SHELLENBERG, A. (1911) Ovogenese, Eireifung und Befruchtung von *Fasciola hepatica. Arch. Zellforsch.,* **6,** 441–444.

SHIBANAI, D. TOZAWA, M., TAKAHASHI, M. and ISODA, M. (1956) Experimental studies on vaccination against *Fasciola hepatica*. *Bulletin of the Azabu Veterinary College, Japan.*, No. 3, 77–86.

SHIRAI, M. (1925) On the intermediate host of *Fasciola hepatica* in Japan. *Sci. Rep. Inst. infect. Dis. Tokyo Univ.*, 4, 441–446.

SHIRAI, M. (1927) The biological observation on the cysts of *Fasciola hepatica* and the route of migration of young worms in the final host. *Sci. Rep. Inst. infect. Dis. Tokyo Univ.*, 6, 511–523.

SIEVERS, H. K. and OYARZUN, R. (1932) Diagnostic de la distomatose hépatique par la réaction allergique. *C. R. Soc. Biol., Paris,* 110, 630–632.

SIMONDS, J. B. (1880) *The Rot in Sheep.* (Reprinted from The Journal of The Royal Agricultural Society of England). John Murray, London, 1880.

SINCLAIR, K. B. (1956) Black disease. *Brit. vet. J.,* 112, 196–200.

SINCLAIR, B. (1960) Serum calcium and magnesium levels in sheep infected with *Fasciola hepatica. Vet. Rec.,* 72, 506.

SINCLAIR, K. B. (1962) Observations on the clinical pathology of ovine fascioliasis. *Brit. vet. J.,* 118, 37–53.

SSINITZIN, D. (1914) Neue Tatsachen über die Biologie der *Fasciola hepatica* L. *Zbl. Bakt.,* 74, 280–285.

SSINITZIN, D. F. (1929) Rediae and cercariae of *Fasciola hepatica* found in water snails, Galba bulimoides techella. *J. Parasit.,* 15, 222.

SSINITZIN, D. F. (1932) Studien über die Phylogenie der Trematoden. *Biol. Zblatt.,* 52, 117–120.

SSINITZIN, D. F. (1933) Studien über die Phylogonie der Trematoden. *Z. Parasitenk.,* 6, 170–191.

SKVORTSOV, A., SMIRNOVA, V. and SISYAKOVA, F. (1936). Récherches sur la morphologie et la biologie de l'oeuf et sur le cycle évolutif de *Fasciola hepatica. Med. Parasit. Moscow,* 5, 257.

SLANINA, L., POPLUHAR, L. and VRZGULA, L. (1955) K terapii fasciolozy oviec, koc a hovadzieno dobytka. *Sborn. Ceskosl. Akad.,* 28, 932–940.

SMITH, W. S. and KEOGH, J. (1953) Liver fluke and black disease in South Australia. *J. Dep. Agric. S. Aust.,* 37, 101–106.

SMYTH, J. D. (1951) Egg-shell formation in Trematodes and Cestodes as demonstrated by the methyl or malachite green techniques. *Nature (Lond.),* 168, 322–323.

SMYTH, J. D. (1954) A technique for the histochemical demonstration of polyphenol oxidase and its application to egg-shell formation in helminths and byssus formation in *Mytilus. Quart. J. micr. Sci.,* 95, 139–152.

SOBIECH, T. (1951) Rozpoznanie motylicy u bydla za pomoeac odezynu srodskornego. *Polsk. Arch. Weter.,* 1, 213–230.

SOGOYAN, I. S. (1955) Pathological changes in experimental *Fasciola gigantica* infestation in sheep. *I Veterinariya,* 8, 155–165.

SOGOYAN, I. S. (1956a) Reparative processes in the liver of sheep after treatment for *Fasciola gigantica* infestation. *I Veterinariya,* 9, 107–112.

SOGOYAN, I. S. (1956b) Comparison of pathological changes caused in sheep by *Fasciola hepatica* and *F. gigantica. I Veterinariya,* 9, 113–117.

SOGOYAN, I. S. (1958) Pathology and pathogenesis in sheep. *Trud. Armyansk. Inst. Zhivotn. Veter.,* **3,** 255–266.

VAN SOMEREN, V. D. (1947) A sedimentation method for the detection and counting of *Fasciola* eggs in faeces. *J. comp. Path.,* **57,** 240–244.

SOMMER, F. (1880) Die Anatomie des Leberegels *Distomum hepatica. Z. wiss. Zool.,* **34,** 539–640.

SOULSBY, E. J. L. (1954) Skin hypersensitivity in cattle infested with *Fasciola hepatica. J. comp. Path.,* **64,** 267–274.

SOULSBY, E. J. L. (1957) An antagonistic action of sheep serum on the miracidia of *Fasciola hepatica. J. Helminth.,* **31,** 161–170.

SOUTHCOTT, W. H. (1951) The toxicity and anthelminthic efficiency of hexachlorethane in sheep. *Aust. vet. J.,* **27,** 18–21.

SRIVASTAVA, H. D. (1944) The intermediate host of *Fasciola hepatica* in India, *Proc. Indian Sci. Congr.,* **111,** 114.

STEENSTRUP, J. J. S. (1842) *On the alteration of generations* (Translation by G. BUSK), *Roy Soc. Publ.,* 1845.

STEFANSKI, W. (1959) Occurrence and ecology of *Galba truncatula* in Poland. *Wiad. Parazyt.,* **5,** 331–334.

STELFOX, A. W. (1911) A list of the land and freshwater molluscs of Ireland. *Proc. R. Irish Acad.,* **29B,** 65–164.

STEPHENSON, W. (1947a) Physiological and histochemical observations on the adult liver fluke, *Fasciola hepatica* L. Survival *in vitro. Parasitology,* **38,** 116–122.

STEPHENSON, W. (1947b) Physiological and histochemical observations on the adult liver fluke, *Fasciola hepatica* L. II. Feeding. *Parasitology,* **38,** 123–127.

STEPHENSON, W. (1947c) Physiological and histochemical observations on the adult liver fluke, *Fasciola hepatica* L. III. Egg-shell formation. *Parasitology,* **38,** 128–139.

STEPHENSON, W. (1947d) Physiological and histochemical observations on the adult liver fluke, *Fasciola hepatica* L. IV. The excretory system. *Parasitology,* **38,** 140–144.

STIEGLER, L. (1954) Untersuchungen über die Zwischenwirtsspezifität von *Fasciola hepatica* L. im Raume Nordbayern. *Z. Parasitenk.,* **16,** 322–350.

STOEBBE, E. (1950) Eine verbesserte Methode zum Nachweis von Leberegeleiern. *Mh. Vet. Med.,* **5,** 295.

STYCZYNSKA, E. (1956) Wplyw wysychania *Galba truncatula* O. F. Mull. na rozwoj i przizywalnosc stadiow rozwojawych *Fasciola hepatica* L. *Wiad. Parazyt.* **2** (suppl.), 261–262.

STYCZYNSKA-JUREWIEZ, E. (1958) Uklad wzystosomawezy pasozyt-jywiciel na warunkow ekologicznyeh drabnego zlwznika wodnego. *Wiad. Parazyt., Warsaw,* **4,** 95–104.

SUESSENGUTH, H. and KLINE, S. B. (1944) A simple rapid flocculation slide test for trichinosis in man and in swine. *Amer. J. clin. Path.,* **14,** 471–484.

SUSUMI, S., KURAMOTO, T. and ICHIHARA, T. (1958) Studies on the rapid flocculation test for fascioliasis. I. *Jap. J. Parasit.,* **7,** 666–673.

SUSUMI, S., KURAMOTO, T., ICHIHARA, TSUYOSHI and ICHIHARA, TRUSUO (1959) Studies on the rapid flocculation tests for fascioliasis. II. Examination for various antigen emulsions. *Jap. J. Parasit.,* **8,** 6–12.

SWALES, W. E. (1935) The life cycle of *Fascioloides magna* (Barri, 1875), the large liver fluke of ruminants in Canada. *Canad. J. Res.,* **12,** 177–215.

SWANSON, L. E. and HOPPER, H. H. (1950) Diagnosis of liver fluke infection in cattle. *J. Amer. Vet. Med. Ass.,* **117,** 127–129.

SZAFLARSKI, J. (1950) Zastowanie proly allergieznej srodskorno- powiekowej w diagnostyce chorob pasozytniczyeh u zwierzat. *Med. veteryn.,* **6,** 585–589.

SZAFLARSKI, J. and NAWROCKI, J. (1951) Zastosowanie frakji wie locukrowej i bialkowej przy diagnostyce motylicy u owiec. *Med. veteryn.,* **7,** 16–19.

TAGLE, I. (1956) Distomatosis hepatica en el ganado. *Bol. chil. Parasit.,* **11,** 35–36.

TAGLE, V. I. (1944) Observaciones sobre la evolucion de la *Fasciola hepatica,* Linneo 1758. Comprobacion del huesped intermediario en Chile. *Rev. chil. Hist. nat.,* **46/47,** 232–241.

TAKASHINO, H., TABATA. H. and KURITA, Y. (1960) Results of investigation of *Fasciola hepatica* infection among cattle at the Higashimatsuyama slaughterhouse. *J. Jap. vet. med. Ass.,* **13,** 209–213.

TAYLOR, E. L. (1937) The revelation of the life history of the liver fluke as an illustration of the process of scientific discovery. *Vet. Rec.,* **49,** 53–58.

TAYLOR, E. L. and MOZLEY, A. (1948) A culture method for *Lymnaea truncatula. Nature,* **161,** 894.

TAYLOR, E. L. and PARFITT, J. W. (1957) Mouse test for the infectivity of metacercariae with particular reference to metacercariae in snail faeces. *Trans. Amer. micr. Soc.,* **76,** 327–328.

TAYLOR, M. (1922) Water-snails and liver flukes. *Nature,* **110,** 701.

TEODOROVIČ, D., BERKEŠ, I. and MILANOVIČ, (1963) Diagnosis of liver fluke (*Fasciola hepatica*) infection in human beings by means of immuno-electrophoresis. *Nature,* **198,** 204.

TEUSCHER, E. (1957) Eine neue praktische Rotationsmethode für den koprologischen Nachweis der Leberegeleier. *Schw. Arch. Tierheilk.,* **99,** 523–528.

THOM, K. L. (1956) *Fasciola hepatica* als Ursache einer Endometritis des Rindes. *Dtsch. tierärztl. Wschr.,* **63,** 389–390.

THOMAS, A. P. (1881) Report of experiments on the development of the liver fluke (*Fasciola hepatica*). *J. Roy. Agri. Soc. England,* **17,** 1–29.

THOMAS, A. P. (1882a) The rot in sheep, or the life history of the liver fluke. *Nature,* **26,** 606–608.

THOMAS, A. P. (1882b) Second report of experiments on the development of the liver fluke (*Fasciola hepatica*). *J. Roy. Agr. Soc. England,* **18,** 439–455.

THOMAS, A. P. (1883a) The life history of the liver fluke. *Quart. J. Micr. Sci.*, **23**, 99–133.

THOMAS, A. P. (1883b) The natural history of the liver fluke and the prevention of rot. *J. Roy. Agric. Soc.*, **19**, 276–305.

THORPE, E. and BROOME, A. W. J. (1962) Immunity to *Fasciola hepatica* infection in albino rats vaccinated with irradiated metacercariae. *Vet. Rec.*, **74**, 755–756.

THREADGOLD, L. T. (1963a) The ultrastructure of the "cuticle" of *Fasciola hepatica*. *Exptl. Cell. Res.*, **30**, 238–242.

THREADGOLD, L. T. (1963b) The tegument and associated structures of *Fasciola hepatica*. *Quart. J. micr. Sci.*,

TÖLGYESI, G. (1958) Über das Verhalten von Kupfersulfat bei Schnecken Tilgung im Gelände. *Acta vet. hung.*, **8**, 17–30.

TRAWINSKI, A. (1959) Diagnostic à l'aide des méthodes sero-allergiques, des maladies parasitaires des moutons, provoqués par les vers. *Bull. Off. int. Epiz.*, **52**, 234–240.

TURNER, A. W. (1928) Le sort des spores de *Bacillus oedematiens* injectées par voie pulmonaire ou intraveineuse. *C. R. Soc., Biol., Paris.*, **98**, 558–559.

TURNER, A. W. (1929) Infectious necrotic hepatitis (black disease) caused by *B. oedematiens* in a cow. *Aust. vet. J.*, **5**, 11–17.

TURNER, A. W. (1930a) Black disease (infectious necrotic hepatitis) of sheep in Australia: A toxaemia caused by a specific bacterium (*B. oedematiens*) in hepatic lesions resulting from the migration of young liver flukes (*Fasciola hepatica*). Aust. Counc. Sci. Ind. Res. Bull No. 46, pp. 1–110, Melbourne.

TURNER, A. W. (1930b) Innocuity and latency of bacterial spores in the animal body, and the factors influencing their development, with special reference to the pathogenesis of black disease. *Aust. Vet. J.*, **6**, 83–92.

UENO, H., WATANABE, S. and FUJITA, J. (1959) Studies on anthelminthics against the common liver fluke. I. Action of four halogenated diphenylmethanes and three diphenylsulphides. *J. Jap. vet. med. Ass.*, **12**, 297–301.

UGRIN, I. N. and SKOVRONSK, R. V. (1959) Fascioliasis in horses. *Sborn. Nauch. Trud. Lvovsk Zooveter. Inst.*, **9**, 219–225.

ULLRICH, K. (1958) Behandlungversuche mit einem parenteralverabreichbaren Leberegelmittel bei Schafen. *Berl. Münch. tierärztl. Wschr.*, **71**, 168–172.

URQUHART, G. M. (1956) Pathology of experimental fascioliasis in rabbit. *J. Path. Bact.*, **71**, 301–310.

URQUHART, G. M. (1954) The rabbit as host in experimental fascioliasis. *Exp. Parasit.*, **3**, 38–44.

URQUHART, G. M., MULLIGAN, W. and JENNINGS, F. W. (1954) Artificial immunity to *Fasciola hepatica* in rabbits. I. Some studies with protein antigens of *F. hepatica*. *J. infect. Dis.*, **94**, 126–133.

VAIVARINA, H. and VIKSNE, V. (1956) *Fasciola hepatica* starpsaimnieka *Galba truncatula* izplatiba Latyijas PSR. *Latv. PSR Zinat. Acad. Vestis.*, **105**, 67–72.

VARMA, A. K. (1953) On *Fasciola indica* n. sp. with some observations on *F. hepatica* and *F. gigantica. J. Helminth.*, **27**, 185–198.

VASILEV, A. A. (1961) Effect of Fasciola hepatica infections of cattle on some of the biochemical properties of beef. *Sborn. Nauchn.-Tekhn. Inform. Vsesoyuzn. Inst. Gelmintologii,* **7/8,** 3–7.

VASILEVA, I. N. (1960) Ammonium nitrate for the control of *Galba truncatula* on pasture. *Veterinariya,* **37,** 41–43.

VERKRUYSSE, R. and DERDE, E. (1959) Onderzoek naar de verspreiding van de leverbot bij het rund in Oost- en West-Vlaanderen. *Vlaams diergeneesk. Tijdschr.,* **28,** 170–176.

VERNBERG, W. B. and HUNTER, W. S. (1960) Studies on oxygen consumption in Digenetic Trematodes. IV. Oxidative pathways in the Trematode *Gynaecotyla adunca* (Linton, 1905). *Exper. Parasit.,* **9,** 42–46.

VESELOVA, T. P. and VELIKOVSKAYA, Y. A. (1959) The use of CCl_4 against fascioliasis in cattle. *Veterinariya,* **36,** 39–41.

VESOLOVA, T. P. and VOROBEV, M. A. (1962) The application of carbon tetrachloride with hexachloroethane against fascioliasis in cattle. *Veterinariya,* **39,** 31–34.

VAN VOLKENBERG, H. L. (1929) Report of the parasitologist. *Rep. P. R. ins. exp. Sta.,* 1928, 36–38.

VODRAZKA, J. (1963) Critical testing of substances against *Fasciola hepatica* in sheep. *Nature, Lond.,* **199,** 96–97.

WADE, L. L. (1952) Effects of low temperature on the eggs of the common liver fluke (*Fasciola hepatica*) in beef livers. *Amer. J. vet. Res.,* **13,** 345–347.

WAGNER, O. (1929) Experimentelle Untersuchungen über die Biologie des gemeinen Leberegels und seine Übertragung auf kleine Laboratoriumstiere. *Münch. tierärztl. Wschr.,* **1,** 28–29.

WAGNER, O. (1935) Hautallergie und Komplementbindungsreaktion bei Trematodeninfektionen. *Z. Immun. Forsch.,* **134,** 225–236.

WALTON, C. L. (1918) Liver rot of sheep and the bionomics of *Limnaea truncatula* in the Aberystwyth area. *Parasitology,* **10,** 232–266.

WATANABE, S. *et al.* (1955) Infestation of *Fasciola hepatica* in *Limnaea truncatula* in Niigata Prefecture. *J. Jap. vet. med. Ass.,* **8,** 290–294.

WATANABE, S. (1958) General review on fascioliasis in Japan. *J. Jap. vet. med. Ass.,* **11,** 293–299.

WATSON, J. H. and KERIM, R. A. (1956) Observations on forms of parasitic pharyngitis known as "halzam" in the Middle East. *J. trop. Med. (Hyg.),* **59,** 147–154.

WEINBERG, M. (1909) Recherches des anticorps spécifiques dans la distomatose et la cysticercose. *C. R. Soc. Biol.,* **66,** 219–221.

WEINLAND, D. F. (1875) *Die Weichtierfauna der schwäbischen Alp.* Stuttgart, 1875.

WEINLAND, E. and BRAND, T. VON (1926) Beobachtungen an *Fasciola hepatica* (Stoffwechsel und Lebensweise). *Z. wiss. Biol.,* **4C,** 212–285.

WELLS, H. S. (1931) Observations on the blood-sucking activities of the hookworm, *Ancylostoma caninum. J. Parasit.,* **17,** 167–182.

WETZEL, R. (1953) Zur Verbreitung von *Fasciola hepatica, Dictyocaulus viviparus, Hypoderma bovis* and *H. lineatum* im Lande Nordheim-Westfalen. *Vet.-Med. Nachrichten, Warburg.,* 133–168.

WHARTON, G. W. (1941) The function of respiratory pigments of certain turtle parasites. *J. Parasit.,* **27,** 81–87.

WIBAUT-ISEBREE MOENS, N. L. (1958) Distomatosis bij de mens. *Tijdschr. Diergeneesk.,* **83,** 877–884.

WIKERHAUSER, T. (1960) A rapid method for determining the viability of *Fasciola hepatica* metacercariae. *Amer. J. vet. Res.,* **21,** 895–897.

WIKERHAUSER, T. (1961) Immunobiological diagnosis of fascioliasis. II. The *in vitro* action of immune serum on the young parasitic stage of *Fasciola hepatica* — a new precipitin test for fascioliasis. *Vet. Arhiv.,* **31,** 71–80.

WIKERHAUSER, T. (1961) Outjecaju rendgenskog zracenja na metacerkarije metilja F. *hepatica. Vet. Arhiv.,* **31,** 229–236.

WIKERHAUSER, T. and BARTULIC, V. (1961) Imunobioloska dijagnostica fascioloze. I. O vrijednosti somatskog polisahardignog i metabolickog antigena za intrakutani test kod goveda. *Vet. Arhiv.,* **31,** 1–7.

WIKERHAUSER, T., BARTULIC, V. and BRGLEZ, J. (1961) Imunobioloska dijagnostika fascioloze. III. Daljnja istrazivanja o vrijednosti mikroprecipitacije kod goveda. *Vet. Arhiv.,* **31,** 263–264.

WILLEY, C. H. (1930) Studies on the lymph system of digenetic trematodes. *J. Morph.,* **50,** 1–38.

WILLIAMS, V. N. (1963) Effect of 4,4′-Diaminodiphenylmethane against *Fasciola hapatica* in the rabbit and in cattle. *Nature,* **198,** 203–4.

WILLIAMSON, K. (1944) The folk-lore of the sheep liver-fluke. *Northw. Nat.,* **19,** 300–301.

WILSON, A. L., MORGAN, D. O., PARNELL, I. W. and RAYSKI, C. (1953) Helminthological investigations of an Argyllshire hill farm. *Brit. vet. J.,* **109,** 179–190.

WINTERHALTER, M. and DELAK, M. (1956a) Tijecenje fascioloze svinja supkutanom aplikacijom tetraklormetana (carbonei tetrachloridium). Prethodno saspcenje. *Vet. Arhiv.,* **26,** 225–228.

WINTERHALTER, M. and DELAK, M. (1956b) Parenteralna aplikacya tetraklormetana (carbonii tetrachloridium). V. Supkutana aplikacya tetraklormetana kad gaveda. *Vet. Arhiv.,* **26,** 299–312.

WINTERHALTER, M. (1961) Mog ucnost luiceny metiljavosti goveda intramuskularnom aplikacijom mjesavina tetraklormetana s parafinkim ili vegatabilnim uljima uz primjenue hija uronidaze. *Vet. Arhiv.,* **31,** 55–70.

WRIGHT, W. R. (1927) Studies on larval trematodes of North Wales. I. Observations on the redia, cercaria and cyst of *Fasciola hepatica. Ann. Trop. Med. and Parasit.,* **21,** 47–56.

YAKOVENKO, P. F. (1959) Carbon tetrachloride against fascioliasis in sheep. *Veterinariya,* **36,** 33.

YAKOVLEV, Y. (1955) An advance experiment in veterinary science — Abstract. *Veterinariya*, **32**, 40.

YAMAO, Y. and SAITO, A. (1952) Histochemical studies on endoparasites. IV. Distribution of glyceromonophosphatases in the tissues of the liver fluke, *Fasciola hepatica* L. *Jikkon Seibutsugaku Ho*, **2**, 153–158.

YASURAOKA, K. (1953) Ecology of the miracidium. I. On the perpendicular distribution and rheotaxis of the miracidium of *Fasciola hepatica*. *Jap. J. med. Sci. Biol.*, **6**, 1–10.

YOSUFZAI, H. K. (1953a) Cytological studies on the oogenesis of *Fasciola hepatica* L. *Cellule*, **55**, 23–42.

YOSUFZAI, H. K. (1953b) Shell gland and egg-shell formation in *Fasciola hepatica* L. *Parasitology*, **43**, 88–93.

YOSUFZAI, H. K. (1953c) Fertilisation in *Fasciola hepatica* L. *Cellule*, **55**, 177–184.

YOSUFZAI, H. K. (1952) Cytological studies on the spermatogenesis of *Fasciola hepatica* L. *Cellule*, **55**, 5–19.

YOSUFZAI, H. K. (1952) Female reproductive system and egg-shell formation in *Fasciola hepatica* L. *Nature*, **169**, 549.

ZAVGORODNI, Y. V. (1955) Subcutaneous application of carbon tetrachloride for fascioliasis in sheep. *Veterinariya*, **32**, 40.

ZDUN, V. I. (1956) The occurrence of *Fasciola hepatica* larvae and their hosts, *Galba truncatula*, under the conditions of the western areas of the Ukraine, S.S.R. *Probl. Parazitol.*, 2nd (1956), 61–62.

ZIOTO, T. (1960) Obserwajce histochemiczne nad rozmieszeniem cholesterolu i witaminy C w konze nadnerczy owice z marskoscia watroly wywolana motylicac watzobowa. *Méd. vét.*, **16**, 646–652.

AUTHOR INDEX

R

SUBJECT INDEX

OTHER TITLES IN THE ZOOLOGY DIVISION

General Editor: G. A. KERKUT

OTHER DIVISIONS IN THE SERIES ON PURE AND APPLIED BIOLOGY

BIOCHEMISTRY

BOTANY

MODERN TRENDS IN PHYSIOLOGICAL SCIENCES

PLANT PHYSIOLOGY